Your Original Health

"The 'Key' To Health Freedom"

By Dr. Wilco

Printed on
"Sustainable Forest Paper"

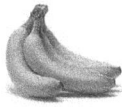

"Your Original Health" Publications
Ibiza, Spain, 2020

** GRATEFUL **

"This book is dedicated to all the people that inspired me to write this Self-help book."

"To all the 'Loving Souls' in my life that encouraged me to pursue my truth."

Disclaimer

The responsibility for any consequences resulting from any suggestion or procedure described hereafter does not lie with the author, publisher, or distributor of this book.

<u>This book is not intended as medical advice.</u>

Copyright Information

Cover Design: *Dr. Wilco*

Copyright © *2020 by "Your Original Health"*

All rights reserved

Second Edition: *October 2020*

You are not permitted to publish, share, or distribute, any of the contents of this book without kindly contacting me first.

Published by
www.youroriginalhealth.com

Table of Contents

Foreword 5
Introduction 9

CHAPTERS

1. Empowerment 15
2. You Are Chemistry 19
3. The Dance of Elements 21
4. Energy 24
5. Nourishment 26
6. Balance 28
7. Step Number One 39
8. Step Number Two 61
9. Step Number Three 79
10. Step Number Four 93
11. Step Number Five 103
12. Step Number Six 111
13. Step Number Seven 123
14. Step Number Eight 139
15. Step Number Nine 147
16. Step Number Ten 159
17. Your Best New Friends 179

QUESTIONS & ANSWERS

– Coffee and Wine	184		– GM Foods	195
– Vaccinations	184		– B12	196
– Superfoods	188		– Sex Health	201
– Satiation	188		– Constipation	202
– Acid Body	190		– Candida	205
– Glycemic Index	191		– Diet Practices	207
– Sweet and Salty	192		– Bacteria / Viruses	210
– Fasting	193		– Why this lifestyle?	216

Foreword

By Dr. Wilco Hermans

It is becoming more and more important these days in this fast world that we claim back what is our given "birthright." And in this book, we will talk about one particular claim, called "Original Health." This is the uncorrupted level of health as it is written in your DNA. The beautiful natural state of your being that only knows how to be healthy.

Do you ever wonder why soo many people are unwell, hospitalized, drugged up, and too frequently need to see the doctor? I believe that it is everybody's right to live a full life of happiness and abundance. Our gift of life is designed to be truly free. In body, mind, spirit, and—freedom of disease.

Misinformation prevents many people on this blue planet from finding and rightfully living their given health potential, what we are all after. And with this exciting level of health comes the power of knowledge. The wisdom to prevent any diseases from getting hold of you, and to give you back your dignity. Accurate and honest dietary guidance is scattered all over the information world and deliberately kept from us. Otherwise, it would be found in mainstream media, studied in schools, and taught in curricula for medical students.

There is no money to be made on healthy people and the *original foods* that will provide this beautiful health. Let's explore these truths here and find the answers to what our natural state of health actually is and how to implement this new information. The time is here for all of us to "wake up" and rediscover our true health freedom, and:

"This book is a good start"

This book is written from the heart, with your health in mind, and I am here to help you with these valuable insights. I want to "empower" you with logical nutritional and dietary support. And these will be pieces of information that you may have heard of but never had the chance to put together to view diet and health from a different angle.

To have your world of *misinformation* shattered before you is certainly not an easy thing to accept, and it takes time and endurance to pursue a new truth. We also need to always question the norms that are the foundations of our societies. The conditioned standards of our lifestyles are presently very shaky as people have started to ask for answers. So, the only real action one can undertake is to seek knowledge. Then this newly acquired information will produce a logical truth that will ultimately set you—"FREE!"

Here in this book, I am setting it up for you. But YOU are the one that has to *free yourself* of your conditioned belief system. That is, when you realize that you are being deceived. You are being told what to eat by the powers of the big food industries that stock the supermarket shelves. You are being misled on what brings you happiness, energy, perfect weight, and real health, which would benefit us all.

So, what is this "Original Health" that the title of this book refers to? Original or natural health, I claim, is the *sexy* state of health of a person. I prefer the word sexy because it sums it all up in one exhilarating word. Of course, all of us have a different notion about what that might be. Thus, the next personal and professional observations on what sexy health is are views that are held by me, but I hope that you can relate and share those with me.

Original, sexy health means that:

- ☆ You get up in the morning and feel bright awake and energized for the day.
- ☆ You are able to do some stretches after awakening and perhaps a brief meditation.
- ☆ You start the day with a fruit meal that will wake up the natural senses and your zest for life.
- ☆ With a straight back you are able to look down to the ground and see your own toes wiggle.
- ☆ You are going positively through your day with a big smile on your face.
- ☆ You have love and respect for our Mother Earth with all the animals on it.
- ☆ You help and support others so that their lives will become more fulfilling.
- ☆ You have that sparkle in your eyes that makes people wonder about who you are.
- ☆ You are confident in who you are being, what you are doing, and are experiencing.
- ☆ You follow a personal exercise program to maintain your fitness level and toned physique.
- ☆ You have vibrant energy all throughout the day until you recharge again for the next.
- ☆ You never fall ill to any type of chronic illness.

If you feel that these *attributes* will look good on you, then I suggest allowing yourself to open up all the "windows in your house," so to speak, and let a new and fresh breeze in.

This new foundation we are about to construct is supported by *ten steps* that will gradually replace your *old structure* with new building blocks. But first, we are going to explore in several pages some intriguing aspects of life. How you are *linked* to your environment through *elements*. And as we are going to talk a lot about these elements of life:

Webster Dictionary's Physics Definition of an Element:
"A small part of the whole. A substance that constitutes all physical matter -- wind, air, fire, water, or a natural environment"

We need to build a motivating positive image of who you are and your place on this beautiful planet. Also, I want to share how everything is connected by a complex intelligence, and that life is indeed very mysterious. So, if you are ready to change your direction and follow a path to better health, energy, and youthful looks, you are definitely ready to read this inspiring book, and to finally:

"Re-invent yourself"

I would like to mention that my person is often present in this book's dialogue. Not that I am eager here to play the *protagonist*, but because I can modestly say that I have experienced a lot. I learned plenty from my own path and other *Souls* on the same or similar journey. I also felt that we will relate better as I genuinely would like you to hear my important message,—thank you!

Introduction

Welcome,

My name is Dr. Wilco, and I am grateful that you found this book (*or did this book find you?*). The knowledge that I am about to share is for all who know that a change is needed and are looking for a logical health path. I am suggesting here to gradually remove health obstacles from your lifestyle in the form of *ten steps*. These will consequently put you on a fast-track to better health. These essential *poor diet/lifestyle* adjustments are my professional recommendations that I hope you will choose to follow. I believe that we all should act from a liberating state that I call "Free Spirit Interaction." Meaning, the influence and freedom of choice that is given to us by the *laws of life*. To act out your entitled rights as an intelligent, free-thinking, and caring human being.

But, the small print reads that you first should have all the information you need before you can make a new conscious decision. How can we make an intelligent conclusion in life if we are not familiar with all the game players of the choice we are about to make? On the one hand, you can say: "That is life, take your chances, go for it!" But then on the other hand, independent research for more knowledge and insights to prevent unnecessary personal damage, it being physical or psychological of nature, could be a better strategy.

When a source of information consists of a decent amount of both commonsense and controversial material and is then objectively studied, you are ready to make that life-changing decision. But the amount of time, or information, that one requires to reach that *point of no return* is different for all.

Some people can read one book or listen to a single person's lecture and feel that every cell in their body resonates with that individual's truth. I would say this sometimes works, but, unfortunately, in many cases, one person's book or lecture is not necessarily the truth spoken, and so, consequently, an unreliable view to follow. On the *other side of the spectrum*, it is also true that many authors are researchers who have taken much time and effort to put sources of information together to form a view, a truth, a philosophy. But still, I am suggesting to you that whatever new interest it is, use the opportunity to research it yourself because honest and unbiased information can still be found in the world when one focuses and researches a particular interest or curiosity. Then, all these pieces of information together will form a more accurate picture. So, make an effort to gather these different opinions and question all the points of view. Then, you are ready for that objective choice you are about to make.

Also, take your time to digest newfound truths. Or, as it often happened to me personally, let the truth find you, which is another position to embrace, for:

"When you ask,—you shall receive"

I am one of these people, by the way. I have *pored* over the same interest, what we as a human race are supposed to eat, since the mid-90s, and this truth-seeking has been challenging to say the least. I am stating here that I have done this job for you. I have done my research to be able to offer people an objective and valuable view of health. But, that does not mean, of course, as I explained, that you should take the word of this author straight away to heart (*especially if you are new at healthy eating and living*).

The knowledge compiled in this book was acquired after years of research, diet trials, and various studies, which led to my PhD. in "Natural Diet and Lifestyle," from the University of Natural Health, USA.

NOTE: I need to point out that I couldn't go in full detail about everything, as this book's size would become way too extensive. So, I bring to your attention the most important aspects, and it is then up to you to look more into it if you feel that you need to know more, or contact me.

This information I am sharing with you here could be a part of your puzzle or maybe the last piece you needed. Clearly, you have an interest in changing your diet and lifestyle, and I hope that my passion for health will become yours as well.

I also would like to mention that I am not the type of health educator that *sugar coats* everything. I will tell it to you straight. I never choose to generalize or judge, but if you feel that I am, then I apologize beforehand. I really would like you to experience this book's dialogue as a conversation between friends. Because at the end of the day, we are all connected. We all are part of each other, and when you are doing well,—I will be too,—and the rest of the world will follow.

It certainly is not easy to change people's belief systems. Most conditioned beliefs are deeply rooted and difficult to shift. I thought about that once while visiting my parents. I was one day together with my dad in the garden removing an old tree stump. It took a lot of digging, wiggling, and even some ax work to convince the remainder of the tree that it was time to say goodbye to the soil that had been nourishing it for all its life (*I truly love trees, but this one was dead for several years*). It takes time before an indoctrinated, and deep-rooted thought system can be removed and updated. The roots go in all different directions, and the deeper they go, the more difficult it will be. It can even hurt at times, the physical and mental notion of letting go, as we are creatures of habit and addiction. We can be so very set in our lifestyles.

It is sometimes said that some folks would change their religion before they change their diet. Specific food items that have been on the table for many years can be tricky to let go of. Food dependencies can be intensely experienced.

Some people out there can leave a habit or addiction, if you will, behind like a bad dream. They take on the newfound information, make the decision, and move on with their adjusted life. Not easy to do, and I was definitively not one of those people. For me, it took time to conform to my new lifestyle and way of eating. Luckily, I had practice over the years with my cooked *Vegan* diet. In the beginning, I often had to say: "No thank you" to various foods that my family and friends thought I was still eating.

When I am talking about adjusting, I am hinting to leave a particular *unhealthy* food item off your plate and replace it with a healthier choice. The biggest challenge here is to leave certain bad comfort foods behind, including spices, salt, textures, smells, and convenience. Plus, the many emotional connections people have with their food, like the special fried curry chicken or meat pie recipe you used to make every Sunday morning with your mom when you were young.

This book is written to help you with this. We will go through these *ten steps* together and confront these changes head-on, as we have to face what we need to battle. Know your adversary and free yourself from its grasp, which is, in this case,—your precious health and life.

This practice is easier said than done, I know, but we will

proceed with *baby steps*, as they say, and you can implement these changes in your life as you see fit. I cannot expect, nor you from yourself, for this to happen overnight as much as you maybe want it to. But the sooner the better of course.

When I became a Vegetarian back in 1990 (*after reading the great book: "Diet for a New America," by John Robbins*) and a Vegan the year after, I was amazed at the attacks on my person about why I would follow this strange *hippie* diet. As animals, after all, are here for our consumption. And even though I was a *strange-one* in other people's eyes, I felt privileged to have obtained a new insight. It felt great to be different and not to be another sheep that follows the flock. I started to read books to learn everything I could about this lifestyle to defend myself and respond with smart comebacks and return questions that would plant seeds and doubts in the *skeptical* mindset of the meat-eater. You can imagine the position I was in as a fresh Vegetarian, but then I became a Vegan, and now following a *Raw Vegan* lifestyle.

There were generally not that many other believers around, in my early Vegetarian days, even none in my social circle. So, therefore, not much public awareness existed and hence little support for my new lifestyle choice. Now, decades later, times have changed thankfully. Even Veganism is growing now exponentially because of increased awareness in diet and health, but we still have ways to go.

I can humbly say that I now have an answer to almost all I am confronted with regarding my diet choice and lifestyle. Not that I want to be some smartass, but it is my job to know. People will defend the *status quo* and want to prove that you are wrong so that they feel less guilty about their choices. It will take time before we all can agree on our diet differences.

Now, many years later, I better understand the struggle for somebody to leave a habit/comfort food behind.

My character will defend a drug user when brought up in a conversation about how bad they are for our civil societies and should be *locked-up*, as some people's flawed view of fast justice goes. Increasingly, more countries now have, at last, a more open-minded drug use policy. Drug addiction should be treated as a health/social problem rather than a criminal issue. It should be controlled and legalized to combat crime.

The addiction to today's foods can be paralleled with drug dependency, and that is what I then present to somebody who judges the drug user a bit too swiftly. But then you continue to open up *cans of worms* because people see the eating of processed foods (*cooked, fried, barbecued, or microwaved*) as a normal act of surviving.

We all are not to blame. Unfortunately, the root cause of this social act is complex and a very extensive subject to write about here. But an important player in this dilemma is undoubtedly the powerful food industry that keeps us: "Happy and content" in our dependency on unnatural foods. They create the addiction, then supply the demand (*hmm, sounds familiar*). There is no money to be made on natural foods. Still, corporations continue to exploit the farmer and the freedom of our seeds. They're aiming to claim the genetic wealth of the planet as their property, by making *open-source* seeds illegal! We must stay alert to these unlawful practices and fight for our foods of the Earth!

I am positive that the reason for picking up this book is because you want to change things in your life. You, as an intelligent person, have become curious about what all this healthy living is about, and you sense that all those medical drugs cannot be the answer. There are all these scary news articles about diseases and people dying too young all around you, and you are starting to worry. You can almost guarantee that everybody has somebody in the family who is not well, to some degree. It's just no fun when you have to make an appointment at the doctor's office that is followed by picking up prescriptions at the pharmacy or being diagnosed in the worst-case scenario. Nobody likes to be or feel sick.

"Nature heals,—the doctor gets paid"

So, take a stand and reclaim what is yours. Take charge of your precious health! I hope that I will succeed in making a more *empowered* person out of you by providing you with this information. My passion and goal are to reintroduce people to the "Natural Hygiene" (**NH**) philosophy, which is founded on nature and is as old as the physical world itself. Its belief focuses on knowing that a *toxic* natural system will inevitably lead to disease, so a *hygienic* clean body is crucial.

I want to share a *Universal mantra* with you to support you on this journey and help you succeed. A profound truth that has been ringing throughout the ages is that:

"Your body is your vehicle for your spiritual experience"

EMPOWERMENT

We all live hectic lives. And in this busy lifestyle, many of us take our health for granted. We rely on our bodies to keep up with what the mind is desiring. We need to work, wash the car, mow the lawn, go shopping, exercise, clean the house, prepare meals, walk the dog, interact with the kids, watch TV, socialize, make love, eat, drink, and then go to bed to sleep to be able to take on those many tasks again on a new day.

That is until you wake up one sunny morning your instincts telling you: "Hey, something is not right." It is usually when that happens (*when alarmed enough after their doctor's visit*) that people decide it is time for a life-change. But normally a person's first course of action is to follow their doctor's advice and prescription that will inevitably lead into a labyrinth of remedies that eventually do more harm than good.

(**Let me state here** *that many medical doctors do great work and are essential for our communities. It is just that they are not schooled in real nutrition and preventive care. They are educated in which chemical drugs go with which symptoms*).

Usually, when all those medications are not providing the cure and/or radiant health that has been promised, people start looking into the alternative route. But it is still a minority who do so because this path is not encouraged by the medical machine. But despite this, the number of people that choose this route is growing. Consequently, alternative treatments are now under threat, as the medical authorities have decided to wage war on alternative therapies and medicines. Certain practices, like acupuncture, can then only be performed by somebody with a medical degree.

This can only mean that they are scared of losing their monopolistic position. This is an alarming situation, and we need to maintain our right to choose our own health path. Doctors do important work, but they are practicing in the dark when it comes to prevention and healing without chemicals.

"Thousands upon thousands of people have studied disease, almost no one has studied health"

- Adelle Davis

I hope that it is clear here what I am pointing out to you. I do not want to overemphasize the not so kind practices of the powerful pharmaceutical companies that want to keep on pushing, through the channels of the medical doctors, the prescriptions of their drugs. It is the darker side of the whole *illness* versus *cure* picture, and I hope that over time more people will wake up to the reality of what is really going on.

Let's talk a bit more about this *empowerment* that I want to teach you. What does this mean? What are these *ten steps* actually for, and what is the end goal or benefit that one can reach when following a cleaner diet? It sounds maybe a bit weird, but that is precisely what you need to change to when desiring a healthier lifestyle. A scenario that often plays in people's lives is the doctor's unexpected bad news of some complications or sudden illness. That is really no fun! It usually starts with subtle signs of discomfort or pain that gradually will form into a full-blown *chronic* condition. A diagnosis can appear like a critical attack on your health. But a *dis-ease* never really comes acutely into your life unless you took a poisonous substance, and your body reacts to the toxic intruder immediately,—as it is supposed to.

Disease happens in an orderly sequence of failure of our natural equilibrium, in the shape of subtle symptoms that will become increasingly persistent enough for warning bells to go off! Maybe not too loud at first, but yet they are *ringing*. The problem starts when people think it is all pretty innocent and will ignore the signs of discomfort, they even shrug it off. If needed, they will try to suppress it with a pain killer, tea, hot bath, or maybe even with a remedy that stems from folklore (*all of which are unfortunately pointless, because only the body can instigate healing,—stay tuned on this*).

I need to share a crucial message! Practically all disease states follow a natural: "Seven steps towards disease pattern." According to the NH philosophy, these steps are always identical in their progression, no matter what condition will be the outcome. Somebody's inherited or created weakness will predetermine the illness that will be manifested. (*the exception here are the uncontrollable events of outside forces, in the form of toxic attacks by animals, pestilence, bugs, or of chemical nature that can poison a person instantly*).

The root cause of most ill-conditions is the over-production of *toxins*, which have a precondition called—"enervation." A continuous production of toxins, which is, to some extent, a normal bodily process, when not taken care of results to a state called—"toxemia" (*meaning, poisons in the blood*). The normal production of toxins by the body is mostly the byproducts of cell metabolism and physical and/or mental stress. These are effortlessly removed by your system and so no real threat. But it is the constant overproduction of toxins that will make: "The bucket spill over," as a figure of speech, and start the gradual poisoning of the blood and other bodily fluids. A satiation of these toxins can/will slowly and surely develop into a diseased state.

These seven steps towards disease are the following:

Enervation ⇒ Toxemia ⇒ Irritation ⇒ Inflammation
Ulceration ⇒ Induration ⇒ Irreversible disease

"Nature is ordered, a sequence of—'Cause and Effect"

And this is where empowerment comes in when you have it within your control to prevent this from happening. You are empowered to the extent that you control your own fate of health without using any scare tactics to make you believe me here. I am purely stating biochemical facts.

YOU ARE CHEMISTRY

All molecules (*two or more Atoms chemically bonded*) of life interact with the elements (*an unsimplifiable basic substance*) within you and your outside environment. Because we are part of everything, and all there is exists as a part of us! And this interaction finds place through the many features of the human body. It would die otherwise (*personally, I always felt that this knowledge should be taught in schools to make kids more aware of life's wonders at an early age*).

This innate cooperation happens through several symbiotic exchanges, namely, Earth (*feet*) Air (*breathing*) Water (*fruit*) Sunlight (*skin and eyes*) Physicality (*touch*) Brain (*emotions*), and our natural foods. All these are essential players of feeling and being human and necessary survival attributes that our body depends on daily to exist.

Let's look at these connections a bit closer:

Earth: .... We connect with the Earth's energies through our feet by walking on its healing carpet (*we need to walk more barefoot to reconnect with nature*).

Air: ...... We breathe in the essential oxygen elements that nourish us and give us life, so pure unpolluted air is of utmost importance to health and well-being.

Water: .... We take in through fruits our essential structured water. Water is life, and so we cannot live without it. We need it for hydration and mental health. Water is the medium we need to center and relax.

Sunlight: . . . Through our eyes we take in the total spectrum of light from the sun to heal, energize, nourish, and support our eye health for endless amazing sunsets. Plus, we absorb vital vitamin D for overall health.

Physicality: .Our body's biggest asset is our skin through which we experience and sense the physical world. Human touch is essential for well-being.

Brain: . . . . . We experience endless emotions throughout the day through biochemical reactions that produce a realization of existence. A response mechanism that enables us to interact within our living world.

Food: . . . . . We eat the energy elements, or called calories, from our natural foods to connect, ground, and sustain our bodies responsibly.

Normal bodily activities, like exercising, walking, standing still, breathing, drinking/eating, thinking, are all biochemical actions. Behaviors that continuously shape us into a human being. This is a remarkably accurate account of what is going on within your body when you are not looking. This survival process runs for you in the background, and it never fails to do what it needs to do to keep you alive and healthy. These processes that the body runs daily are incomprehensible,—in complexity and in number.

"Disease is just health malfunctioning"

By this I mean that your body only knows the state of health, and it is inherently programmed to be just that. Being sick is unnatural, and so the exact opposite state of health, a sign that something went awry. It goes against all the *laws of life.* Being ill is the result of a health imbalance. When respecting these natural laws, your bodily functions can continue backstage undisturbed without you ever having to worry about any ailments coming your way. Here is where you decide if you want an abundance of health and energy, or prefer to gamble with your well-being. Or put dramatically:

"To play Russian roulette with your health and life"

The great law of life states:

"Every living cell of the organized body is endowed with an instinct of self-preservation. Sustained by an innate force in the organism called 'Life Force' or 'Nerve Energy.' The success of each living organism, whether it be simple or complex, is directly proportional to the amount of its life force and inversely proportional to the degree of its activity."

THE DANCE OF ELEMENTS

As I explained, we process the elements of the environment through our body's organic systems to exist. This is clearly a marvelous intelligent system that makes life truly a dance of elements. Interestingly, WE cannot survive without nature, but Earth herself will do fine, even thrive without us.

There is a crucial factor involved here that plays a key role: "instinct." We depend on instincts for our survival. All the swimming, flying, hopping, or walking creatures in the world follow their natural given instincts.

There are many different types of behaviors that influence our lives and those of our fellow creatures on this amazing living entity we call our home. But we will, in this book, only explore the "Eating for survival" part. Our original foods play such an important role here because when our symbiosis with nature is intact, you are linked, and become—"ALIVE!"

We are part of a very intricate cycle, the *cycle of life*. And we have a purpose to play out in this living merry-go-round. If you are aware of it or not, we are all made of the same stuff (*animate matter*) found everywhere where life exists. It can be difficult sometimes to get our heads around something this profound. It is also a head-spinner and easy to forget that we are *floating* in space (*but in orbit*) on this big blue ball in an immense complex Universe. Filled with *particles* that are the foundations of life. It is truly magical!

So, let's travel from space back to our food because we will need to rebuild if you are looking for a better health path. Groundwork needs to be constructed, because what is a house without a solid foundation? We need to be able to withstand impacts from all directions, meaning, when you become an outsider (*although animal-free diets are finally becoming acceptable now*) you will most likely be questioned, like I was, about your new diet choice. I always suggest taking these encounters with a grain of sea salt and approaching these discussions with a sense of humor and understanding. Learn from my mistake. I often acted too defensively around animal rights, and these emotional skirmishes will not serve you.

In 2001 I joined a nonviolent Vegan protest against animal cruelty in San Francisco, and we were met with unbelievable hostility. And so in return, I found myself acting aggressively at these pro-meat supporters! Very regrettable, I see now.

> *"In a gentle way,—you can shake the world"*
> – Mahatma Gandhi

Whenever I can talk to a group of people, I always ask two questions first. "Who loves food? Please raise your hands." Predictably all hands go up. "Who wants to be healthy?" Also here they go up. These responses are no surprise as we all want the best of both worlds. Of course, the challenge lies in combining those two, to find a way to have real health and enjoy the foods on your plate. To accomplish this, we need to take on these objectives:

1) Eliminate all the diet obstacles in your life that are preventing *your original design* from surfacing.

2) Allow your natural eating instincts and bodily functions to return after completing objective *one*.

3) Adapt your life to the *laws of nature* that allows you then to eat deliciously and remain healthy.

Our own body and mind's *original state* is obstructed. It is hindered in being what it potentially could be. Most people go about their daily business and feel that they are healthy, and I sincerely hope for them that this feeling is accurate. But the interpretation of health is different for every person. Many, I have learned, convince themselves that they are. Some people can only accept that they are sick when they are forcibly bedridden and cannot do anything other than rest. This is the ultimate plea to force the body to stop,—to go into *lockdown*! To conserve energy, so it can initiate self-healing.

Symptoms of not feeling well are not always recognized as a real problem. As I said before, they are often ignored and/or suppressed with some medication that works like a band-aid. The *wound* is covered up, and the *bleeding* stopped, but the cause is not addressed. The wound can even *reopen* again at any time and could come back with a vengeance.

ENERGY

Energy is the most precious asset that we have! Physical, mental, and spiritual energy. What is having a lot of money in the bank when you are not well? To maintain health, we need to have energy, which is not hard to obtain because it is already given to us as much as we need.

We are all born with a set measure of energy, and each individual has variable allocations for their energy storage. More specifically, everyone's energy stores are differently utilized, depending on various aspects, like diet, lifestyle, and an individuals predisposition. Whatever the case may be, we are given a sufficient sum of energy for organ function and movability to survive in our natural environment. Energy is created by the brain, which then runs our organs (*more on that later*). And to be able to feed ourselves, we need to move our muscles/body to seek out food sources.

In nature, we also have all types of animals with different strength and energy levels. Some animals have prolonged energy throughout the day, and others only a powerful burst of energy that will provide them with sufficient agility to get their meal for the day. The larger cat species are a great example of animals that chase their prey for a short period and display incredible strength and speed to catch and kill their dinner. Afterward, these hunters are totally incapacitated. Because they have a large stomach volume, it is no problem for them to tear off and gulp down large amounts of flesh. All their energy then goes to digesting, and the animal will sleep until hunger strikes again.

Then there is the antelope, in many cases the catch of these cats, which pretty much eats only grass, foliage, and leaves.

These animals can easily not only run fast for large distances if needed, but also outrun a large cat if not old, too young, or wounded. They have a prolonged energy reserve that is required for their survival in the wild. Most antelopes are grazers (*some are browsers*) and have four stomachs to handle plant fibers. Because of this, they have a less natural energy drain than, e.g., lions and leopards. Who again, need plenty of time to digest their meat, despite having strong stomach acids (*PH 1-2*) and short intestines to assist their digestion. It is also very interesting to know that large cats, or similar predators, always go first for the stomach contents. They know instinctively that these herbivores have in their stomach the essential plant elements that they nutritionally need. Then, for dessert, they go for the other organs because they are also nutritiously valuable. It is a beautiful symbiotic relationship despite appearing very violent and cruel.

We humans also fall in a category. We belong to the family of animals that need to consume foods for prolonged energy. Like apes, we are primates, given all the physical attributes (*opposable thumbs*) to harvest the foods that we biologically need. Foods that we not only digest easily and nourish us, but also enjoy. More on this later in *step* number one, but I feel that it is already clear that we are not naturally invited for dinner at the home of Mr. and Mrs. Lion.

"Instinctively,—we are not meat eaters"

If not convinced of this fact yet, then please read on as we will further explore this topic and other dietary truths that will change your present beliefs. I really urge you to research this yourself, but please be always aware of the meat industries propaganda lies that are found everywhere.

Besides the suggested removal of meat from your diet, this book will give you *nine* other *steps* to promote better health for an improved and consequently a *sexier* you who is presently hidden under the layers of wrong information. Take these *steps* at your own pace. Don't be too strict on yourself too soon if this information is totally new to you. Most people need time to apply changes in their diet. Be kind to your self. And if you "Fall off the wagon" at the neighbor's barbecue party, just try again and do better next time. Build your belief system first and then start to act upon what you have learned.

NOURISHMENT

I always let people know that I am not the type of educator who showers people with boring statistics. There are more than enough writers doing this already. It is still good though to once and a while look them over. Proper data is important, although I have learned that those can have a degree of unreliability. We live in a world of deceit where powerful control is exerted by companies that pursue their agenda.

So, I personally prefer to tap into people's logic. Waking up their instincts and talents for reasoning bestowed to any human being with a reasonable amount of intelligence (*I do see the challenges a person can face these days, as there are so many conflicting theories*). A vital ingredient here is to permit yourself to be open to new knowledge that can possibly shake you at the core. Then your feelings (*this is your Soul talking*) will decide your next move. What do you have to lose? You can always go back to your old routines if it does not resonate with you over time.

"Whatever satisfies the Soul is truth"
                                                                            - *Walt Whitman*

One of the many pieces of the food puzzle that needs to be scrutinized is *proper nourishment*. What are the foods that truly nourish you? After all, we need to sustain ourselves for survival. This is a vast subject and needs to be looked at from many angles. But I feel that it is all pretty simple really, it is a matter of basic chemistry.

As you now know, the body interacts with its environment, and this environment is made up, like your body, of elements, of the particles that form all life. We come or are born from these same elements that exist all around us, and this beautiful interconnected relationship defines us as a species. We are literally created from all the elements that surround us, that we live in. That's why it is so essential that we eat elements that are in a recognizable and so usable form that we can only find in our natural whole food sources.

> **"There is nothing that can be found in the Universe, that cannot be found within our bodies"**

And vice versa. I deeply love that truth. It really fascinates me the complexity of it all. So, what is required to sustain and nourish yourself? For one, we need calories, as you probably know, and calories are also called "energy units." To be able to take in these calories we need to eat. Eating is the most important way to provide these essential units to the body. Besides our food intake, there are a few other controversial means (*briefly covered on page 19*) that also partly nourish us, like the practice of Sun-gazing (*energy fed to us through sunlight*), barefoot walking (*energy emanating from Earth's surface*), and disciplined breathing techniques (*nutrition obtained through Prana*). Unfortunately, we cannot explore these here because of the extensiveness of the subjects.

Many of us just love to eat! We also enjoy standing in the kitchen to prepare the meal that you have been craving all day. Eating is an enjoyable cultural practice and what's on people's plates varies from nation to nation. But no matter how different these meals all over the world are, we all need to eat for *nourishment* to have *physical energy* for survival. It is indeed very interesting to see these different eating habits on our globe, as I have had the privilege of observing several. But as you can imagine, it has gotten out of hand. The actual purpose of nourishing with our life-giving foods has been replaced by the pleasing of the palate.

One reason (*more on this later*) for us *falling off the path* is that when we eat a food that we like, we stimulate a part of our brain (*endorphins kick in*) that tells us that we want more. This area of the brain is indeed a teaser as it is naughtily designed to experience pleasure. These pleasurable sensations will then routinely develop into behavioral addictions. So, the apparent innocent indulgence most of us find in food triggers this euphoria of happiness. This is where we unknowingly "corrupt" our given pure instincts when consuming unnatural foods. Sweet sugar, especially, is a need, a pleasure, and an addiction, all under one hat. Which, if not correctly guided, will lure you into a health dwindling loop, as we will learn.

BALANCE

Life is about the balance between *Yin and Yang*. This mystical equilibrium maintained by your body's intelligence needs to be at all times in sync with all the other elements. What is required is the whole package, and the word *whole* cannot be expressed enough. When food comes directly out of nature, preferably straight from the tree, it is whole. It is a perfect food that consists of all that we need for health and well-being,—this is how it is designed!

People continue to worry (*besides the protein*) that they do not get their daily doses of vitamins and minerals. This is a fear that not only exists because it is common knowledge we need them for health, but also because it is a creation by the supplements industry. I have encountered articles stating that today's vegetables and fruits are nutritionally insufficient. That we need to supplement our diets! These are ridiculous false claims so they can sell more *overpriced* and *pointless* supplements to you.

And where do protein and fats come in? I hear you ask. These are equally important to your diet but in surprisingly low amounts. Fats and proteins are present in all fruits and vegetables in various quantities and in their most usable biochemical form. It is often not understood that we need to consume *amino acids* that the body forms into valuable protein. The body needs 20 different amino acids to function (*nine we cannot synthesize and need to get from our diet*). Even though animal proteins are a complete protein source, they require too much effort from the body to process. Plant protein is, in that way, superior, and so our better choice.

Let's sum up the requirements for true unconditional health:

- Energy, for the sustaining of bodily functions.
- Foods that are recognized by the chemistry of the body
- Foods that are properly digested and create no toxins.
- Foods that produce an alkaline environment.
- Foods that have their water content intact for hydration
- Foods that contain all the essential nutrition.
- Foods that bring forward a healthier environment.

Let's explore these requirements in more detail for you:

Energy, for the sustaining of bodily functions.

Natural energy or *nerve energy* is an electrical current generated in the brain. It feeds and links all the organs and functions together. It is our battery for proper functioning. Therefore, we need sufficient natural energy that will assist in removing toxins and other tasks within the system.

When a body is *enervated*, an efficient removal is not achieved, and an accumulation of toxins is slowly formed. A drained system will start to *save* important bodily tasks for later when it has a renewed energy storage to deal with the imbalance. But when this enervation is not corrected, those critical tasks will not be completed, and the body's natural equilibrium will become compromised. Toxemia is inevitable. Only when a healthy abundance of energy is present can the body prevent a buildup, and so avoid—"self-poisoning!"

All organs work together for efficiency. The human body contains eleven major organ systems, like Cardiovascular, Respiratory, Nervous, and Digestive system, to name four. When not enough energy is present, the weaker enervated organs will be supported by the stronger ones. But this life-sustaining organ collaboration will inevitably fail and produce more demand on the system. Hence, more enervation is created, and self-correction becomes very difficult.

The only way to properly regenerate energy is by *deep REM sleep*. When a clean natural diet (*less digestive energy loss*) with exercise (*creates healthy tiredness and stamina*) and a healthy amount of sleep is maintained (*uninterrupted sleep with dreams*), we will have balance and plenty of energy reserves. Then, energetic health becomes—first nature.

Foods that are recognized by the chemistry of the body.

All life is chemistry. To maintain a balance with nature is essential for pure health. The elements that make up your food need to be assimilated by the chemistry of your body. These life-giving elements become distorted when changed in any way, like cooking, barbecuing, and microwaving. Their chemical structure will become *alien* to the body and so set aside to be dealt with later. Only to form toxins in the end because the body will never be able to properly handle these *estranged molecules*.

In essence, the integral structure of our whole, fresh, natural, and uncooked foods are already the components you are made of, as these elements exist all around us in nature. It becomes then no effort what so ever for the body to fully assimilate and make these molecules/elements of your food become a part of you. The cycle is complete when your fecal waste *(ideally from a clean raw diet)* will nourish the soil that grows the delicious fruits that you will then eat again.

Foods that are properly digested and create no toxins.

When whole natural foods are consumed, there will be no conflict with assimilation, and no toxins will be created. Adulterated or processed foods, on the other hand, will create digestive conflicts as they cannot be properly assimilated. So, when a natural clean diet is followed, one eats fairly simple and avoids wrong food combinations.

When the protein, fat, and carbohydrate elements are indiscriminately combined together, digestive trouble can/will occur (*in concentrated form only, as these three are contained in small amounts in most natural foods!*).

Proper food-combining rules (*explained later one*) with a sequential eating routine (*page 100*) will need to be followed to avoid stomach battles. Only then can we manifest complete digestion with no issues. Food needs to travel in the shortest possible time through our long digestive tract. Luckily, the natural water and fiber contents of our *original* foods will assist in this task. When all is in order, we would neither hear nor feel our stomach and have odorless digestion.

Foods that produce an alkaline environment.

Besides breathing, an essential and challenging task for the body is to keep our blood at a slight alkalinity of pH 7.4. (*potential Hydrogen*). This is important because otherwise, we would simply die. The body can handle an over-alkaline environment better than an over-acid one, so we need to keep our blood and other bodily fluids clean. Blood nourishes the whole body. Our nutrition is delivered through the tiniest of capillary blood vessels, so then you see that these delivery channels need to remain unobstructed. Our saliva is alkaline and contains the primary carbohydrate digesting enzyme called *Salivary Amylase*, which points to an interesting hint to what our natural diet actually is.

To produce good quality and nutrient-rich blood, it has to be low in fat molecules and contain our natural food nutrients. All cooked foods, therefore, produce an acid body, especially animal products. All whole fresh fruits and veggies, as you can guess, results in an alkaline system (*page 190)*. Nuts and seeds, however (*essential now in your new diet*) produce mostly an acid reaction, and therefore need to be minimized.

The acid/alkaline ratio will be in the safe margins when you keep it at 30–70%. Cell metabolism also produces acid ash in the body, but it is hardly a task to eliminate this from the system when sufficient energy is at hand, as you learned. Citric foods (*despite being very acid*) oxidize into *carbon dioxide* and water, resulting in an alkaline body. But I don't over-consume these as I still feel the acidity effect. So, make sure you always chew properly and mix the food with your alkaline saliva. Do not gulp down an acidic fruit juice!

Foods that have their water content intact for hydration.

The human adult body is about 60% water. (*various organs are even composed of more, or less, water*). Our brain's water content can even be as high as 85%, so we cannot survive without water and need to always stay hydrated.

Water is the natural medium for all cells. It lubricates, connects, and is our transport for nutrients (*blood plasma*) and waste. Talking about bodily water, we do not *pee* enough, and it is a problem. Cooking removes the valuable water from our foods that we have to replenish again through drinking.

Fresh produce contains plenty of water, and this H_2O compound hydrates and helps with digestion, as it stimulates the peristaltic muscle movement of the bowels. And together with the fiber, it guarantees a quick digestion and disposal of our daily accumulated waste, which results in a clean body. I would like to see any person attempting to clean their home, car, or themselves, without water. Same here, we cannot effectively clean our systems without it. Water is also an element with many mysterious properties (*see water step*).

"Water is the driving force in nature"
- *Leonardo da Vinci*

Foods that contain all the essential nutrition.

We are all worried that we do not get enough vitamins and minerals in our diets because we all know that we need them for good health. True. We also know that we destroy most of those with the practice of cooking, but this does not seem to worry people enough. Not everything gets killed, some nutrients may survive, but all elements, as we learned, work together. When some essential ones are missing, crucial biochemical bonds cannot be created. The body needs the *whole family* to truly benefit from assimilation.

Many modern-day products on our supermarket shelves contain added minerals and vitamins. These appear to be good selling tactics from the manufacturer, but it is only a desperate and necessary act to put some usable nutrition back into their product after they have removed all nutritional value of any kind. But these added nutrients can be questioned regarding their usability. These are fragmented elements and do not constitute a wholesome and fresh natural food where all the elements are intact. You will get all the nourishment that you need by eating a whole and unadulterated alive diet.

Fruits, all veggies, nuts, and seeds contain enough nutrition for you and your family to enjoy radiant health.

Foods that bring forward a healthier environment.

You are a natural environment that exists within another environment, and both are symbiotically linked together. When a farmer maintains his land with love, uses freshwater, preferably plants heirloom seeds, and does not pollute with chemicals, he will produce a good and healthy crop. The opposite farming practices, together with aiming for mass yields, will produce a sick and nutrient-poor soil over time that will be reflected in his crops. The soil he depends on for his livelihood will become more and more polluted and will slowly die. He will try to save it in time with more chemicals from the agricultural industry that promises him just that. Maybe for a short time he will be saved, but still, the end result will be dead soil and no crops (*crop rotation, pioneered in the early 16th century, is the solution here, together with chemical-free farming, to prevent nutrient-poor soil*).

Agrochemical products are the equivalent of throwing gasoline on the fire! They will make things eventually worse than it was. And this destroying of healthy farming conditions can be compared with our body's environment.

"When you pollute the environment around you you will inevitably disease your own"

Animal husbandry is unnatural, and therefore unsustainable. It causes the pollution of our water, soil, air, and your body eventually. Only the growing of healthy organic produce with intelligent "Permaculture" philosophies (*farming practices implemented with the balance of nature*) will keep the soil clean and nutrient-rich for endless quality farming. Support this worthy and essential cause for our future.

"Eat organic!"

All you hear about these days is the lessening of your carbon footprint to heal the environment. Electric cars are part of the solution it is said, and they are a step forward, but if you genuinely want to help to minimize the impact of *carbon dioxide* on the world, becoming a Vegan is a much better solution because of lesser cattle dung (*methane, ammonia*), water pollution (*the use of antibiotics and other chemicals*), and deforestation atrocities (*burning and cutting down our lungs of the Earth for cattle grazing*).

And as we are on the topic, *plastics* have infiltrated our environment in the worst possible way! Plastics in our rivers, lakes, and oceans is one thing, but we are presently also dealing with *microplastics* that are found in foods, and now even in our rainwater and airways! Our many decades of looking the other way and ignoring Mother Earth has now come to haunt us as we are now suffering the consequences of our lack of responsibility!

We as a world are too slowly coming together to combat the issue, so it is presently an impossible task. The billions of tons that are dumped annually in our environment is an alarming number and real solutions, in my opinion, are still far away. The recycling, innovations, and awareness in our western countries are leading the way to solutions. However, without pointing any fingers, there are still too many nations where the attitude and desire to help are falling behind.

Five Asian countries are named as the worse polluters of discarding plastics and other destructive environmental trash into their rivers that eventually will end up in our oceans. Somebody ring the alarm bells, please!! But the local people are not to blame. It is the government's responsibility to set up programs, recycling industries, and take care of education in schools and to the general public.

We now ban plastic grocery bags, great! But what is the point when we still see soo much fresh and processed foods wrapped in plastic, and at times on foam trays? A practical no-plastic solution needs to be found soon, together with a world-over agreement to ban it finally from our planet.

A much needed caution:

I would like to end these *food requirements* with a caution that is tied in with all the previous food suggestions. This warning is expressed without the creation of *fear*. I personally do not like the deliberate fabrication of fear, as many people do so they can sell their views more easily. I come from a place of caring for your health.

So, what I am referring to are the many incidences, often fatal, of—"food poisoning!" Food from an animal source (*meat, poultry, shellfish*) that is not well prepared or bad can become potentially dangerous. The chances of you becoming seriously ill, or die, from these food bacteria than from a fruit or vegetable that is off, are many times higher. You will be loading another bullet to play Russian roulette with your life! "Do you want to take these chances?"

So, please be aware that these animal-based foods need a lot of special care. They need refrigeration, freezing, heating, and be eaten within a specific time frame because decaying animal matter is a bacterial nightmare. To me, this is a logical indication that we need to stay away from these food sources. Choose your food supply wisely as your health comes first.

So, are you ready for your new path?

It is time to dive into the "ten steps." Let's have fun exploring these suggested diet changes. Again, give yourself the time to revolutionize your life, which can be scary and difficult at first, but when a new and healthier you will be the outcome then,—isn't it all worth it?

* * * * * *

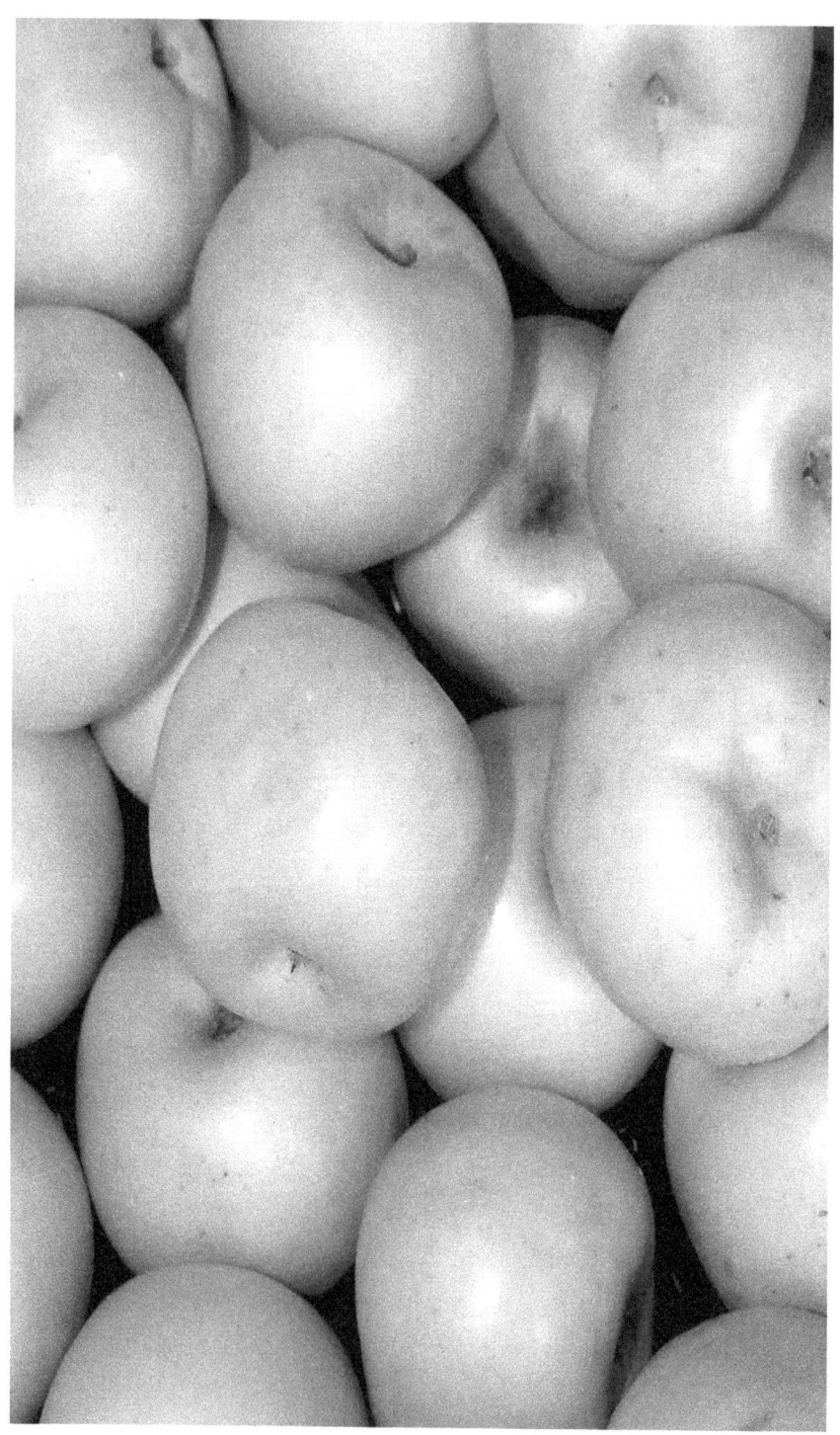

STEP
NUMBER ONE

MEAT

We are going to enter the world of meat. I will take you on a journey to show you what it means to consume the number one food choice in our modern and primitive civilizations. I will share with you valuable truths and different perspectives. This is crucial so that you can make up your own mind about this very first food item that is advisable to remove entirely from your life. Remember, knowledge is empowerment!

So, let's start at the beginning, kinda. Before there was any sign of what we would call civilizations, early man relied on meat for its survival, as they learned that animal flesh would sustain you longer. Not surprisingly, because our ancestors and all cultures throughout history ate meat it is seen as proof that it is our natural food. Also, since the *ego* was invented, meat has this idea of *strength* around it. You are a man when eating meat, a leader, and this dogmatic view is difficult to remove as it has been ingrained in our societies ever since.

The meat industry has been using its skilled marketing strategies for decades to keep the illusion alive that we benefit from its consumption. But their costly propaganda campaigns these days needs to be continuously "beefed" up to stay effective, which is no surprise because more and more people are finding out the truth. So, . . . then what is this truth?

The discussion usually grows from the fact that man once was a hunter and gatherer. He lived in an era where he would kill anything that moved and then would share this prize with his family or people from his tribe, no argument there (*of course, in some of our present day's primitive cultures, this is still the way of life*). The same as you cannot argue that mankind was also surviving once, before his hunting days and discovery of fire, on mostly fruit and certain grasses. Which is a very probable fact as well, as we will see.

Throughout man's history, meat consumption was also seen as a reflection of wealth. You are successful when you can supply your family or guests with a slab of meat for dinner. These days though, the meat industry has created a market where meat prices have gone down dramatically. Meat is available to anyone who wants to eat it. Regrettably, we are now paying a very high price for its low market costs through the loss of health and our environment's destruction.

Interestingly, in his famous book: "The China Study," Dr. Colin Campbell, who conducted the most comprehensive health study ever done on large populations, revealed that various cancers would fall mostly on well-off families in poor countries that could afford—meat and dairy.

In 1959 they found in Tanzania a very important skull. The owner of this skull, who lived about two million years ago, was named the *Nutcracker man* because he had these large flat maulers that clearly were used as a tool. It was assumed that they were utilized for the crushing of nuts and other hard objects. These finding's final conclusions differ, but most archaeologists seemed to agree that this nutcracker man did actually not eat nuts as his or her staple food. But it consisted primarily of fruits, grasses, and certain plants called sedges.

In another interesting report by Dr. Alan Walker, a well-respected anthropologist (*May 15, 1979, New York Times*), it was discovered through electron microscopes that there was practically no wear on the teeth enamel of this prehuman or *Hominid*. They were even highly polished! Meaning, they did not eat any meat because it contains bones and those leave scratches. Dr. Alan Walker even exceeded the astonishing previous nutcracker man hypothesis by stating that they ONLY ate fruits! Because plants and grasses also leave traces on the enamel, from silica crystals, and fruits do not contain them. So, does this conclusively prove that this very early man was a Vegetarian? No, . . . but most likely he was. But despite all these insights, the controversies still continue.

So, what are you missing out on when NOT eating the flesh of innocent animals?

Let's start by telling you that the meat will hold and contain various toxic substances at the moment of slaughter that you inevitably will consume. And that will be Adrenaline, Uric Acid, and Creatine, together with the toxins of the animal's metabolic waste that resides in the muscles. The poor animal knows it is about to die and so its adrenaline level will shoot up and will flush all throughout its muscles. In other words, animal fear is created, and—fear—is being consumed. Fear is a very negative energy that should not be taken in by us and, most certainly, not from another lifeforce. Fear will also go through the antelope body we talked about earlier when it is about to be eaten. But of course, these large predators are not affected by this killing as we can be.

Do you see yourself, by the way, like a lion, chasing an antelope? Can you envision, if you happen to catch and kill one (*no guns and knives allowed*), to tear it open with your bare hands and teeth and dive straight into its guts and enjoy the blood, hair, and other gore to your heart's content? If we are designed to eat meat, then this is how we should enjoy it. Nature does not provide us with an oven or barbecue and a fancy sauce to go with it. It does not serve it to us on a plate, all neatly cut, fat and bones removed. It is true, of course, that some primitive cultures out there in the world are still hunting for food, even with spears and machetes (*large heavy knives*), but they only kill what they need and will cut the organs out, instead of eating it there and then. Understand that they also prepare their meat with fire, as it is pretty indigestible in a raw state because our human physiology is not suited.

So, for many people, these hunting scenarios are proof that eating meat is normal, that it is a natural food source. I will agree that it appears this way. One important difference between primitive cultures and the western world (*besides our convenience of buying it and kitchen rituals*) is the disrespect we have for an animal and paying somebody else for killing it (*when you purchase meat, this is what we do*).

What follows is that our guilt-free meat is being packed neatly in plastic that we then find in the supermarkets next to the choices of condiments to make the bland tasting meat savory. These convenient unconscious practices indicate an important fact! We are totally disconnected from our foods! Where it comes from and how it is produced. So, when we put all these meat buying conveniences to the side for a moment, then a simple respectable truth emerges:

"When you want to eat it,—YOU should kill it!"

But besides the ignorance of where all this flesh comes from and what it takes before we find our ribs and sausages in the meat section, most people still have no clue about another essential truth. That there is a link between *health* and *food*.

People still think that we can eat anything that our eyes feast on. There is plenty of physical proof that we just can't digest meat properly, and you have already learned that complete and fast digestion is very important for vibrant health.

We lack the important enzyme *Uricase* to help break down the high amounts of *Uric Acid* found in animal meats, which is an extremely acid-forming substance. So, we have then acidic urine, with feces and pus, that is being held in the flesh. Meat lingers in your system for a very long time. It putrefies, or plainly said, *rots*, and creates toxins because it has no water or fiber to help it along through the system. Try to picture this to have a real effect on you.

When *Creatine* first was discovered, it was believed to be essential for strong muscle development and necessary in our diet. The debates around this theory continue as some say it is harmless, while others warn of its dangers. It is still praised by athletes and bodybuilders as an enhancer, but it comes from an animal's muscle and really has no place in our bodies. Finally, more and more athletes are now opting for plant-based meals to support their performance.

What is truly inspiring is that we see more competing *strongman* in the world following a Vegan diet. They are not only breaking records of strength and endurance, but also the myth that you need to eat meat to be strong. I have followed a great and passionate muscle man, Patrik Baboumian, who won many titles, like Germany's strongest man in 2011. This is where we are heading, and I love it!

To continue, due to bacterial decomposition, the flesh starts to rot the moment the animal dies and will continue to do so until it is eaten. In the slaughterhouses, they let the animal breakdown deliberately for a while so that the enzymatic process can proceed in *predigesting* the meat for you for more tenderness. Chemicals are used to give the flesh that has started to turn *black* a bright red and bloody appearance for the consumer's appeasement. Sadly, many animals are also diseased. The factory farming procedures make an animal weak and prone to many maladies, which makes sense considering the living conditions they're found in. Many are not even inspected or treated, as it costs too much time and—money. So, the malignant tumors and other conditions will land on the plate of the consumer. "Bon Appétit."

Parasites Anyone?

Another issue with eating meat, especially pork when undercooked, is favoring the conditions for a parasite to grow (*Trichinosis*). This is soo gruesome to even write about, but it needs to be brought to your attention. I remember cases in the news of people contracting a brain parasite after eating unsafe meat. The thought of this creature settling in your brain tissue or making a home in your intestines is a horror story to me, and I am sure to you too. They thrive in acid conditions and unclean environments. So, let me list a few symptoms that will suspect you of housing a trespasser and then seek a way to evict this/these unwanted guest(s):

- Unexplained constipation, diarrhea, or persistent gas.
- Unexplained rashes, eczema, hives, and itching.
- Constant hunger, even when you are eating enough.
- Muscle and joint pain.
- Grinding your teeth during sleep.
- Itching of the anus or vagina.

I feel that we can stop at these insights as I do not want to gross you out too much. The next danger we need to bring to the table is the cooking of the meat. Oil of some kind, which is a concentrated fat, will be heated up first until it sizzles. Then, the animal's meat, also high fat, is fried in the pan (*animal meat is high fat even when it is sold as tender or lean*). So, we have a lot of fat to deal with here. Fat elements can/will become dangerous food particles that cannot be underestimated. This will become evident when any type of fat gets heated up to very high temperatures. The heating will cause a dangerous change in the molecular structure and be formed into what we call: "Maillard molecules" in the meat's fat. Another issue when it comes to frying oil or even grilling meat are the "Hydrocarbons and Free Radical Fatty Acids." These naughty boys are most definitely *carcinogenic* and eventually create an *unsexy* toxic you. You will agree that this is not what we want.

Also, when you are *NOT* eating any meat you will miss out on the smörgåsbord of chemicals that the animal took in over its lifetime in prison. These man-made poisons with their high toxicity level injected in these animals for growth-*enhancing*, disease-*preventing*, and flesh-*preserving* (*for after slaughter*), are just baffling. Meditate on that one for a moment.

Let's review the facts around the consumption of what we call a "happy cow." This is a cow, pig, lamb, chicken, or any other farm animal, that has been given the dignity of open spaces. It is allowed to graze in the field and live a relatively normal life. Some animals munch on the nutritious green grass, and others are fed natural feed, and so are kept clear from any chemicals. The idea is to raise them as they did in the "good old days." The meats coming from these farms are branded organic and are preferable if one really needs to eat meat. The picture of farming animals for food does improve a lot, but we still have to deal with the fact that animal meat is way too fat. An animal that can roam around and is not fed horrible *growth enhancers* is leaner, of course. However, lean meats can still be too fat (*10 to 20 % per 100 gram*), and fat calories per gram are little over double (*9*) than from protein (*4*) and carbohydrates (*4*). What also doesn't help is that fat stores toxins easily, and you remember that they need to be removed from your system as quickly as possible.

An alarming number of people are overeating on fat and protein, and overconsumption of these, strangely enough, promotes even more eating of them. It is imperative to know that when eating nutritionally poor food, the body will start to crave even more food because of its need for valuable nutrients. And so the perpetual cycle of compensating for the poor nutritional intake with even more poor foods begins.

The excessive protein intake that comes with meat-eating is a significant burden on the organs in general, specifically on the liver and kidneys. They cannot handle the excess when eating a happy cow or a factory one. When eating organic meats, you are still taking in the high cholesterol, uric acids, and some of the other attachments that I mentioned earlier. Plenty of people are aware of this but do not see them as a threat to their health. They still trust the fact that cooking destroys everything, so the food then becomes safe to eat.

To the followers of the—"Paleo diet." If somebody claims that eating raw meat is part of our natural diet, this person needs to be told to put away the salt and sauces because nature does not provide these for him. He will need to eat the flesh as it is, but he could pour some extra warm blood over it to keep it juicy. I know that there are individuals who have no problem with this, but how can you enjoy that, and for how long? If they eat meat this way to prove a point, they will not act very logically. To remind you again, the practice of eating cooked or raw meat also includes the killing of the animal.

How come some people are capable of taking the life of innocent creatures without flinching? One is because the brutal practice has been a part of their culture for generations. Or, they are farmers and got accustomed to slaughtering. Or perhaps, it is their daily job, and they have become mentally desensitized. It is most certainly not proof that we are inherently designed to end an animal's life against its will!

And when a life is taken, you will have to prevent the meat from contaminating. As again, meat, or any other animal product, will go bad very quickly and become dangerous to eat. You are not allowed to put it in your freezer as Mother Nature never created those for you to use (*exceptions exist, of course, like when living in the unnatural arctic regions of the planet and you can store the meat in ice*). But of course, a hungry and inventive man in desperate need to conserve his bloody catch through the seasons discovered the practices of *smoking* and *curing* meat to prevent bacteria growth.

Please ignore the fact that many animals are eating other animals as that is their evolutionary instinct, and it is none of our business. We are not designed to do the same. Talking about design, here is a small excerpt from the "blueprint" of life. All creatures, big or small, are part of a fascinating organic system, guided by instinct. The innate diet behaviors of all living species are rooted for survival, and therefore, they follow the complex laws of life. This way, we all can maintain an equilibrium in the food sources on our planet.

Nature is perfect and all the answers can be found within:

CARNIVORES ⇩	HERBIVORES ⇩	FRUGIVORES ⇩
Animal has claws and walks on all four legs	Walks on all four legs with hooves	Walks upright, has two hands and feet
Sharp and pointy teeth shaped for tearing of flesh	Teeth shaped for grinding grasses and leaves	Teeth and jaw shaped for biting and chewing soft foods
Salivary production is low	Salivary production is high	Salivary production is high
Acid saliva and urine	Alkaline saliva and urine	Alkaline saliva and urine
Intestinal track is 4 times body length	Intestinal track is 18 times body length	Intestinal track is 12 times body length
High stomach secretion of hydrochloric acid	Weak stomach secretion of hydrochloric acid	Very weak stomach secretion of hydrochloric acid
Secretion of Uricase is high. Is needed for breaking down of uric acid,	No Uricase production	No Uricase production
Have round stomachs	Special stomach compartments	Stomach with duodenum
Survives on flesh	Survives on grass, leaves and plants	Survives on fruits and vegetables

On a side note—These different diet behaviors ingrained in each animal can become corrupted in certain situations, like a lion in a zoo or circus. It is then not only stripped of its instincts to hunt for food, but it is also fed dead inferior foods that don't provide its complete nutritional needs.

Happy news from your author—The awareness towards captured animals is slowly changing. Circuses are showing signs of closing down as increasingly more countries are now prohibiting the use of live animals for entertainment. Also, the zoos seem to lose their popularity. Courts have started to rule that animals are sentient beings and that they have rights, like dolphins, whales, and elephants. But what is frustrating to me is that most civilized nations have laws in place that will prosecute anybody abusing a dog, geese in the park, or kill kittens, but intelligent pigs and gentle cows are left behind!

I would like to ask of you to never again, if you ever did before, to pay for any type of animal show. Besides zoos and circuses, places like aquariums, Seaworld's, and safari's that need to be boycotted and closed down. We need to restore our animal's natural habitats that are slowly disappearing. All creatures, like us, desire to be "FREE!!"

Animal Atrocities

I am sorry if you feel maybe that I am going on about this. But I need to add a few more crimes inflicted upon our animals, besides the cruel caging and slaughterhouse displays, so that you will be fully informed about animal abuse.

FOIE GRAS—This dish is consumed by French cuisine lovers. It is the horrible act of FORCE-feeding ducks and geese to create enlarged livers to be eaten as a pâté. I dare anybody who is a frequent eater of this dish to watch the videos that show this cruel practice.

ALCOHOL—Somebody came up with the idea to feed alcohol, beer, and wine to cattle for flavor and tenderness. This is also a cruel idea and should be made illegal yesterday.

Please try to read these other atrocities we commit to our *friends* and then check how you feel about them:

- > Cutting off tails and beaks
- > Ripping out teeth
- > Removing their babies
- > Pumping them full of drugs
- > Depriving of sunlight
- > Stealing milk from mothers

Then let's also not forget the countless LABORATORY experiments performed on animals so that we can have safer beauty products. This has to really stop, and you can help by growing awareness and shopping sensibly. Thank you!

Possibly, you are also asking: "What about fish?" I cannot recommend the consumption of fish either. The general rule is to stay away from any food source that has or had a face. Fish is a muscle with fins made out of fat and protein, and because it has no fiber, you can forget about a fast passage. People still see eating fish as a healthy option, but I am sorry to say that this is not true. Fish flesh is also too fat. Depending on the fish, it is usually in the 40-70% range (*which will become even fatter when fried in oil*). Too much fat is a threat to your health, as you are learning now, and later on.

Another issue related to eating high-fat foods is oxygen deprivation. High fat and protein diets cause the blood cells to stick together, called the "Rouleaux effect." The result is less surface area so that these cells cannot deliver the same quality and amount of oxygen so that you can breathe properly. And isn't that one of the precious gifts of life, to be able to breathe and live? Where is the logic in hindering the body's system so that it cannot function to its full capacity?

Cholesterol levels are also too high to consume safely. And on top of all this, eating fish creates a very *acidic* body, a concern that I will keep on raising in this book. An over-Acid system will promote osteoporosis (*more on this later*) and a playground for bad bacteria and viruses. An *alkaline* system is our healthy predisposition, and we should not challenge this natural state. So, . . .we gotta leave fish off our menu.

Also, in this day and age, we need to highlight the dangers of chemicals. The oceans and everything in it are polluted! So fish are *toxic* and become dangerous to eat (*fish farms are equally bad*). Microplastics, mercury, and other pollutants are now found in our sea life. Ohh, what a mess we are in.

Other inhabitants of our precious oceans are the crawling sea creatures that are boiled alive in pots and served on a plate for our pleasure. It is just insane and cruel. And then we have the many shellfish options that are consumed raw as a delicacy. These are yet another round of playing "Russian roulette" with your life. People have died repeatedly from eating ill-prepared shellfish. It is just not safe to eat them. Did you know, by the way, that the intelligence of *octopus* can surpass the intelligence of your pets? These are the more sentient creatures of our oceans, together with dolphins, orcas, sea otters, and our majestic whales, to name a few.

On a special note—For me, if there is one necessary reason to stop eating fish, it is to STOP the fishing industry! The destruction they cause with their nets on the ocean's delicate Ecosystem is just criminal. Our aquatic worlds are being overfished for decades now. We need to stay out and let its equilibrium restore itself. I have seen the secret footage where they needlessly slaughter dolphins, sharks, and turtles, caught in these nets and useless to them,—cold-bloodedly!!

Let's get back to the meat.

Then the fact again that meat does not contain any fiber. Because of the lack of fiber, water, and the very poor stomach secretion of hydrochloric acid, you cannot really assimilate animal flesh. It will linger in your system until it starts to putrefy in your pristine digestive track. Where is the logic in doing this to your health once you have learned this?

But the most significant indication that we are not designed to eat animals is the psychological part of our humanity,—our mental disposition. To face an animal, look into its eyes and then kill, skin, gut it, and then deal with all that blood and stench of death to then be served raw or cooked for dinner is clearly not in our nature. But this bloody scenario could apply and be justified (*maybe*) when we don't have sufficient natural food at hand. When our lives depend on it, our survival instincts will overwrite our emotional ones. We will kill when truly starving (*but with our eyes closed*).

People, unfortunately, murder other human beings, even regularly. Generally, these sick individuals are emotionally scarred, get generously paid to do so, and/or are plain insane. PDSD (*Post Dramatic Stress Disorder*) is a growing concern among our brave, "conditioned to kill" soldiers. The high numbers of suicides in the military *(suppressed news)* clearly show that the act of killing can *haunt* a person for a lifetime.

A hypothetical experiment would be to put a starving child (*because children have their natural instincts still intact*) in a closed environment with a rabbit and an apple. Everybody knows that the kid would eat the apple and play with the bunny. There is just no way it would be the other way around.

So, we can only come now to one conclusion.
When NOT consuming any meat:

You are not missing out on anything at all!

As a matter of fact, you will become more humane. You will become a "real respectful citizen of the world" when caring for our Earthly creatures and our environment. You will not partake anymore in the destruction of pristine jungles that are being burned/chopped down and used for the grazing and breeding of animals for burgers. Your *Aura* will become brighter and more colorful. Your positive energy will attract more beautiful people into your life, and the negative energy of death from eating your fellow-creatures will disappear.

What is fascinating to me is that I hear people comment a surprising number of times: "But plants are alive, how do you justify that?" Every time I wonder where people get this from. Not that I disagree, because I read a most intriguing book published in 1973, called: "The Secret Life of Plants." I learned from that controversial book that plants, besides having some kind of sentience, are here to nourish us. Fruits and greens would otherwise wither away when not eaten, and so their purpose in sustaining us would be missed.

See the beauty of all animals on this planet, even the dangerous ones, like crocodiles, sharks, tigers, and bears. Leave them be. They have their place in nature and the same right as you to be here, the right to raise their own offspring and feed them with the foods they are designed to eat.

To sum it all up, you will become a, "sexier human being" in all aspects when respecting all life. Now, if this is not a true cause, then what is?

Mankind though still has a long way to go. We are far from living harmoniously with all creatures. Please decide now to become a part of this change that we need. Your love for meat is a poor relationship, as it does not love you back. It will cause a slow decline in your health, your—Original Health.

What do you choose?

I read some interesting articles about companies that research the trends for the future. And when it comes to the "future of foods," these well-respected businesses are seeing the direction of a complete food market overhaul. They are predicting that the meat and dairy industry, as we know it, will be pretty much non-existing in 15 to 20 years (*no doubt that in the lesser developed countries, it will take longer*). Plant-based alternatives are now gaining serious market value. Cultivated meat is another option, as some people will always want to eat cow and pig. These are created by in-vitro cell culture of animal cells, called "cellular agriculture," so no more meat from slaughtered animals!

This is what the dictionary says about "Carnism,"

"**Carnism**—the invisible belief system, or ideology, that conditions people to eat certain species of animals. Carnism is essentially the opposite of veganism, as 'Carn' means 'flesh' or, 'of the flesh' and 'ism' refers to a belief system."

What can I do now when not a Vegetarian yet to switch to healthier alternatives? I am happy you ask. Luckily, our first world countries have a plenitude of food options as great health markets and stores are showing up everywhere. When you start looking into the possibilities, you will be surprised by what you can find. Even regular restaurants now have delicious Vegetarian and Vegan options, so give them a try.

I will include in every *step* alternatives for you to eat when in a transition state, for when you are new at this and need to slowly adjust to this exciting new lifestyle. I will also finish each *step* with my *cleaner* advice for people who want to go all the way. Take your time to get used to your new routine when eating out or playing chef in your own kitchen. Also, don't forget to compliment yourself so now and then for what great health changes you are making.

So, if you ate meat yesterday and say, "NO more" at this moment, then I applaud your decision and have the transition suggestions coming up for you that will slowly wean you off this *No-No* food. I will keep these suggestions short because there are many Vegetarian/Vegan cookbooks and websites out there. Join a specific social group that can help to keep you going. There is a sea of inspiration out there.

When in Transition

The best way to begin is to slowly exchange your meat dishes with a Vegetarian alternative. If you feel that you cannot do this overnight, then take one meal at a time at your own pace.

We are living in a fantastic time to be or become Vegan. These new companies that are supplying us with amazing alternatives to meat have just outdone themselves. There is now a new generation of innovative food technologies that hopefully will change our food choices and sources. We now have plant-based burgers that look, taste, smell, and even bleed (*beet juice*). Since 2016 we find these in supermarkets meat section because these alternatives are not exclusively created for Vegans, but actually the meat-eater (*hence the fake blood*). The market knows that eating animal meat is a dying trend and eventually unsustainable, so a new market needs to be created. So, with all these new advancements, you do not have to miss out on anything at all.

"Eat respectably and with love for a clear conscience"

Social gatherings and family parties are one of the biggest challenges that you may face. I have heard this frequently that people do fine at home until they are invited to a social function and do not dare to *inconvenience* the host. Stand your ground, dare to be different! Brave the jokes from your coworkers and your uncle John. Come prepared, and just put your veggie burger on the barbie. Practice comebacks in your head just in case you need to educate aunt Gertrude if she asks you: "How come you are eating so weird?"

If you pay attention to the news and especially the Vegan channels, as the regular ones do not cover these topics, you will learn that in the world of celebrities, many are turning Vegan. Singers, politicians, athletes, movie actors, etc., are all catching on. Now, how is that for a solid piece of information to enlighten people with? Whatever you do, believe in why you are doing it. When you believe in something, you should stick to it, as that is one of the privileges of being free. No need to do what everybody else is doing. YOU are the one in charge of your health.

An argument that is out there is that a big guy (*or woman for that matter*) can never go Vegan. A true misconception! Patrik Baboumian, who I mentioned, is a big guy and who will tell you that it is possible through eating sufficient valuable calories. Many big people carry a lot of fat and water and when they would switch to a plant-based diet, they would become healthier, leaner, and possibly stronger as a result.

All the Hercules's out there know that muscle is built through weight resistance exercise but are brainwashed into thinking that you only will have the power to do so by eating meat. A brief warning about *protein* powders is needed here!

The most famous example of the animal kingdom that Vegans use as hard evidence is the male "Silverback gorilla." Those boys can become a whopping 180 kilos (*400 pounds*) of solid muscle purely by eating (*a lot of*) plants.

My Cleaner Advice

This cleaner advice that I will be ending every *step* with are my stricter suggestions if you are thinking about following an even cleaner lifestyle than a regular Vegetarian or Vegan diet. I understand that it is not an easy goal, as these diets are strict enough for many. But still, I praise anybody who chooses an animal-friendly path. We all make our decisions based on not only our *addiction* and *will-power* levels, but also with what we are most comfortable with. So no judgment there. But I still would like to suggest to you here to venture out to the cleaner side once in a while,—as you might like it.

When you decide to eat now as clean as possible, eating alternative meats is not really recommended either. These are great transition foods, but ultimately these foods need to be heated and contain salts, spices, and preservatives. At the end of the day, these foods are also not whole and fresh. Even though they're not animal products, they are still considered "dead food." Try to incorporate more fresh greens and fruits in your daily diet. Snack on nuts and seeds, enjoy an avocado (*soak your nuts/seeds for easy digestion and to remove the "Phytic acid," together with grinding for better assimilation*).

Because your body has been cleansing all throughout the night, it will be a healthier morning routine to start the day with a *break-fast* of colorful juicy fruits. A bowl of bananas, fruit smoothie, or a few apples will fill you up, clear the mind, and energize you for the remainder of the morning. I know you are thinking: "That will not sustain me, I'll be hungry all the time." Be patient. In time your body will adjust and then uses this pure nutrition to maintain a satiated you. The goal is to feel and be lighter. But until then, what helps is to drink water when you feel hungry and have no access or time for food. Keep always in mind that it is often beneficial to abstain from eating so that you can practice,—"intermittent fasting."

Try also to minimize the tofu dishes and other alternatives because these are also processed foods. Rely more on pulses, like beans, lentils, chickpeas, to consume a superior plant protein meal. But better yet is to switch to higher quantities of clean alkalizing fruits to fill you up. Take your time to make this transition. You will be amazed when your taste buds start to experience those real original flavors again.

I need to give you a heads-up here as the eating of lots of fruits concerns people, so there is a persistent myth to tackle. People worry that all that fruit sugar will make them gain weight. Glucose (*the simplest form of energy for the body*) not utilized by the body will be converted into fat. This is true, but this goes for all sugars. So, the *key* here, of course, is "EXERCISE!" A lazy body that is not burning any calories (*glucose energy*) becomes less equipped to burn fuel and stores it when the body is not exercised. The "mitochondria" in your muscles (*the more muscles, the more mitochondria*) processes the glucose and fatty acids from your diet and storage. Where there is muscle, there can be no fat!

I need to stress again that protein is found in all foods, so also in fruits and vegetables. Of course, the protein amount is much less than in animal products, but you are learning here that we don't need that much protein to survive and thrive. Therefore, sufficient quantities of greens and fruit together with small daily amounts of "nuts and seeds" will be enough to maintain, strengthen, and control your healthy weight (*these always in conjunction with exercise*).

Eat accordingly to your personal needs. An example would be a bowl of lentils, beans, or chickpeas, with greens and an avocado. When wanting to eat clean, four to eight bananas, a small whole watermelon, or a six-pack of apples, with spinach and avocado (*after 30 min.*). Fruit sugar is your pure fuel that will keep you going, and some fat will support your strenuous activity. A new Mantra for you to take in is:

> **"When you eat enough calories, you will get enough protein"**

Special Attention—The cleaner you decide to eat, the more detoxing you will stimulate, and so the more withdrawal or cleansing symptoms you might experience. Depending on your level of *toxicity*, your body will have to go through these. You are experiencing more toxic removal than usual because you are clearing the way for this to be possible. This is definitely a good thing. This is the indication that what you are doing is working! For this reason, it is for very toxic people a better option to slowly remove a *step* out of their life. Symptoms range from feeling slightly nauseous to mild and severe headaches. These body discomforts will gradually disappear over time, and the new healthier you will surface.

* * * * * *

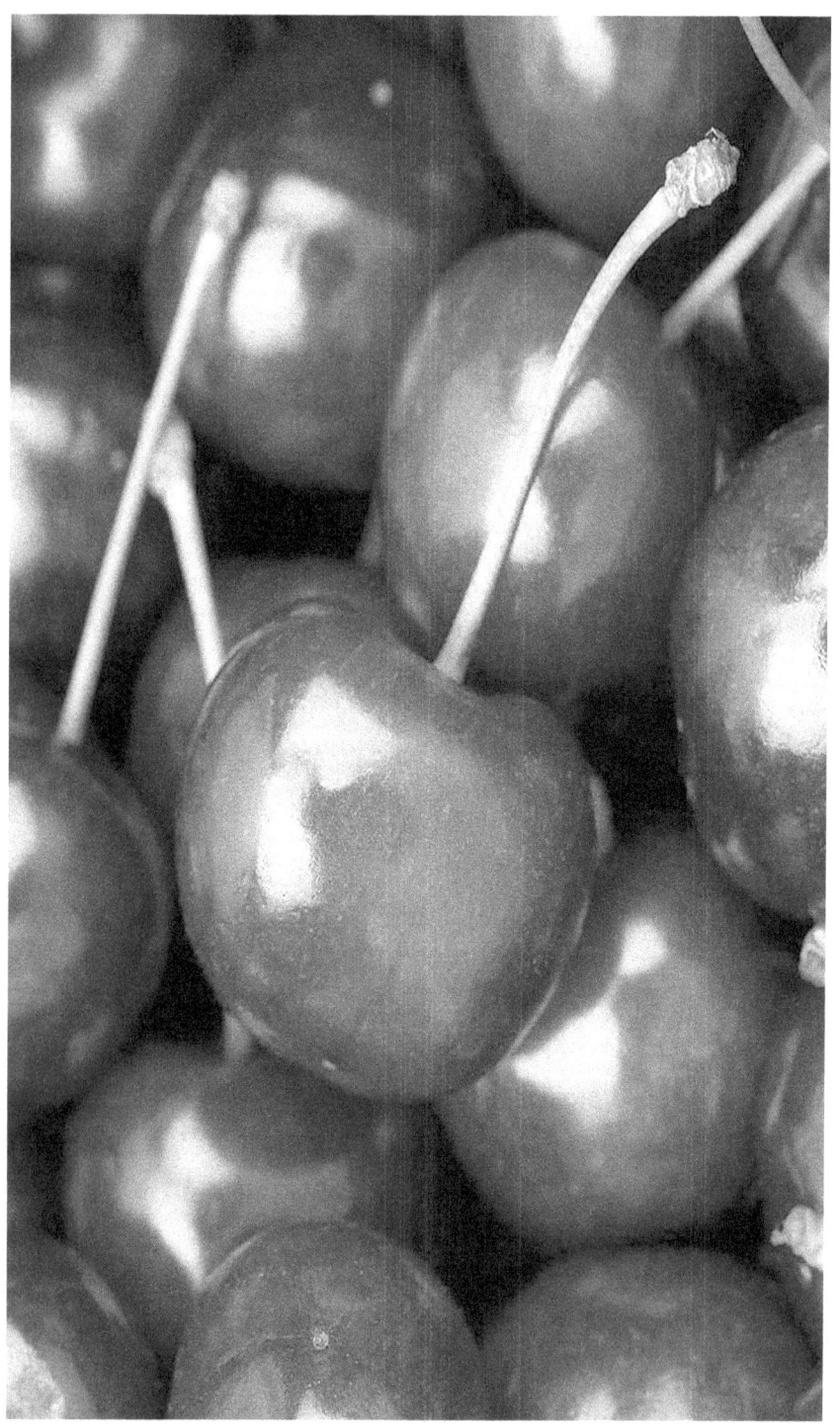

STEP
NUMBER TWO

DAIRY

I would like to start by inviting you for a nice walk. We will wander into a lovely green grass field where we have a couple of happy cows grazing in the sunshine. Cows are very curious animals, and it is known that they even like classical music. But a lot of people do not think too much of a cow. They feel that it is a stupid animal with the sole purpose of giving us milk, meat, and shoes. But a cow has a role and place in life and a right to exist. It feels pain, fear, emotions, and wants to love and care for its young as we care for our babies. And the milk that this mammal produces is only meant to be for that purpose,—to feed its baby.

We feed our babies with human milk, and it is one of those wondrous moments between a mother and her child. The milk that our beautiful mothers produce is a source of incredible nourishment that a wee one needs for early development. Preferable for as long as possible (*2-3 years*) so the child will get the right start in this amazing thing called "LIFE."

Most of us still respect the feeding mother in our social environment, be it on the subway, at the doctor's office, or in the park (*in some cultures, unbelievably, it is still a taboo*). If we could only respect the cow as well, or any other nursing animal, then a giant leap towards peace with the animals would be made. They all deserve the right to live, love for their young, and their feeding process. And each nursing mammal produces milk exclusively for its offspring.

Cow's milk has a different composition to human milk. The milk of a cow contains much more protein and ours more carbohydrates. The baby cow is pretty much straight on its hooves after being born, but WE love to linger in our mother's arms. Not only because we like it that much, but also because we have no choice. We develop, in comparison, very slowly. The protein or casein that is high in cow's milk will support the baby cow's fast-growing bones. For that, the mother cow has a simple and monotonous diet that consists of grass and hay, it is her source of protein. Grains are not part of the staple of a cow's natural diet but only fed to them for quicker fattening (*the grain issue will be explained later on*).

This eating of only grass will deliver constant quality milk in contrast to human breast milk that is very susceptible to the mother's diet when she eats a variety of foods when nursing. Nature intended for human milk to be watery and sweet at first, to become more creamy later on to satisfy the babies appetite better due to increased calorie requirements. The makeup of our mother's milk is foremost carbohydrates, fat, and then protein. The milk of a cow is predominately protein (*casein*). The unborn calf in the womb is already developing strong bones so it can walk within a few hours after being born. It should therefore not be fed to a human baby's fragile frame because cow's milk is simply "bovine growth liquid!"

A high protein intake is a huge stress and toxic to our organs. Protein poisoning can create various sensitivities in babies, and later on in life, like allergies, colds, diarrhea, and asthma. Picture that delicate and *pristine* digestive system of a baby and what damage is being done in that early stage of life when nursing with cow's milk, as many new parents do. When a mother is not able to breastfeed, other options exist.

Our first development lies in the brain, as we are more complex. And as the brain needs blood glucose, it becomes obvious why we have more carbohydrates in our first food than anything else. Clearly, we are born with a sweet tooth.

We do not need as much protein as is commonly believed. This myth is endlessly brainwashed into our everyday life: "We need protein to be strong and survive!" Nothing could be further from the truth. We do need protein (*more specific, amino acids*), no doubt there, but the required amounts are low. We need first simple carbohydrates to start developing our brain, then more sustenance, like fat, for further complex developments. Next, more protein, to grow our skeleton frame so that in between 9 to 12 months (*varies from child to child*), he/she can start making its first steps.

An analogy I use often is that when you start building a house, you need bricks, but when the house is finished, it will be pointless to keep on hauling in the same amount of bricks (*protein*). A few for repairs to keep the structure intact, yes, but not an excessive amount every day. Just imagine the large piles of unnecessary bricks collecting at your front door, blocking your daily activities.

When the calf reaches a certain point in development, it becomes weaned off the milk, and it will start to eat grass. It will stop drinking its mother's milk. All mammals are doing it this way,—why are we not? Why do we keep on drinking milk and on top of that from another species? I hope you see that this practice is ludicrous and understand that we keep drinking it because we are told to drink it for our bone health.

Okay, get this, America is one of the highest consumers of dairy products in the world, and yet, over 44 million suffer or will be suffering from *osteoporosis* in their lifetime. Plus, it is not an elderly condition anymore as it is shifting to younger ages now. You would think that if the message were valid, there would be hardly anybody left, in any nation, with the dreaded bone weakness,—makes sense, yes?

   The propaganda machine surrounding all dairy is very powerful and has been pumping out misinformation for many decades now. If we do not stop this obfuscation of facts, we will continue to suffer ill health because of it. So why are the masses being deceived? Easily explained,—money. The advertising corporations representing the dairy industry are continuing to brainwash the populations that milk is good for you. It is a multi-billion valued industry. A most famous and classic, yet devious, ad campaign that went around the media circus was the "Got Milk?" images (*for people not familiar with the ads, they involved images of celebrities wearing a "milk mustache," promoting dairy consumption*). Presently, they play the innocent card of cute farm animals grazing in the sunshine, and a farmer working hard for that *quality* milk that you and your family deserve to consume for great health. Do not be fooled by these scams.

   Animal milk is far from the common idea that it still is: "Nature's most perfect food." Animal milk is, for most people, indigestible. If no symptoms occur in the infant or teen years, then they could manifest in adulthood. The poisoning effects of milk can result in cramps, diarrhea, bloating, and gas. All over the world, 75% of the populations are mild to severely intolerant to dairy, an amazingly high number. We need "Rennin and Lactase" to be able to properly digest and assimilate milk. After the young age of three to five, we will stop producing these necessary enzymes to digest our mom's low protein breast milk.

If you have undigested particles in your pure system called "estranged molecules," that will wander around your body without a purpose and acidify the system,—they will become *toxic*! You need to avoid these toxins at all costs because toxemia is the precursor and root cause of all ill-conditions. Poisons first saturate the bloodstream and bodily fluids, then, the cells, tissues at the cellular level, organs, and systems.

When animal milk is consumed, the bacterial flora will decompose it and ferment and putrefy the milk, with toxins as the byproduct,—not good! Of course, the body, with its infinite intelligence, has a defense against this assault. It will start producing more mucus that acts like a wall against this toxicity. Consequently, this excess secretion can manifest in the common cold, asthma, sinusitis, and even bronchitis, all respiratory eliminations. The body uses the quickest exits at its disposal to do away with these violations.

I will honestly tell you here that since I turned Vegan, back in 1991, my attacks of frequent colds stopped. I had that from my Mother, and she still gets colds with the slightest draft because her defense system is constantly irritated (*work in progress*). Remember the "gradual steps of disease?" My personal health does not contain any colds anymore, and you can also eliminate these annoying periodic sniffles, or worse.

"We need calcium for strong bones." Very true, but you're not going to get these strong bones from animal milk. I have to possibly shock you here by revealing that they even become weaker because of it (*this explains the high incidences of osteoporosis in today's dairy consuming world*). The body needs to *buffer* the acid condition that is caused by dairy consumption by using alkalizing calcium. And where is this calcium found? In our skeletons! It is *borrowed* from our bones, but never *paid back* when you continue to create an overly acid system. And so another perpetual cycle is born.

    The milk that you find in the supermarket is pasteurized. Louis Pasteur thought in the 1800s that he would be doing the world a favor by inventing the pasteurization process so that foods would have a longer shelf life. My oh my, if he only knew. Yes, commercially, it is of tremendous benefit, but the food value merely goes down the drain, so to speak. When any milk is pasteurized, the calcium becomes unusable to the body (*modern research dismisses this theory, but Vit. D is, to this day, still added to milk*). The molecular structure becomes distorted and, therefore, unrecognizable. It becomes totally pointless to drink or eat it. The milk protein (*casein*), high in cow's milk, becomes coagulated and hardened, and the body does not know what to do with the stuff. Plus, the coagulating process, or *curdling*, will continue to obstruct other usable food particles present in the stomach and render them useless as well. And so a ripple effect is created.

    Did you know that they manufacture wood glue and other adhesives out of casein? This sticky element is not intended to be inside our pristine bodies, and it does not stop there. When the estranged calcium molecules of the pasteurized milk cannot be absorbed by the body, it deposits them in the soft tissues of beautiful you creating "calcification." This can lead to severe obstructions and well-known conditions, like "arteriosclerosis." Your thousands of tiny capillaries, some even hair-thin, deliver valuable blood nutrients to the tissues. Blood flow removes any impurities and excess out of the tissues to get filtered out by the lungs, kidneys, and liver. What do you think happens to your biochemical marvel when this essential delivery and cleaning system gets clogged up?

We have not even touched upon the dangers of antibiotics and other diverse chemicals given to these animals. Why do you think that many children and adults are unwell and/or overweight and suffer allergies? The verdict is still out, or rather still kept from us, on what the consequences will be over a longer period of time, but the effects are here today.

Many people encourage the consumption of goats, sheep, or even camel's milk and are hailed as the solution. I think that these other kinds of milk are preferable to cow's milk (*not factory farmed*), and fresh raw milk is superior to any pasteurized milk, and it doesn't matter from which animal. But, when it comes down to the hard honest fact, all animal milks are inadvisable to consume. This is how the dictionary describes a poison:

" [1] A substance that through its chemical action usually kills, injures, or impairs an organism. [2] Something destructive or harmful. [3] An object of aversion or abhorrence. [4] A substance that inhibits the activity of another substance or the course of a reaction or process (*a catalyst poison*)."

Perhaps it seems harsh to brand milk as a poison, but this is precisely what animal milk is to us. One could argue that we have been drinking animal milk for thousands of years, and we have adapted to its foreign composition. But when you look into *malabsorption* research, it confirms that this has not happened. The numbers all point to the fact that various cultures suffer allergies from dairy. It varies from nation to nation, but there is no indication that it is globally tolerated. As also revealed in: "The China Study."

When animal husbandry became a way of the masses, as people lived apart from their natural food sources and had to secure food, milk became the nourishment for millions. It was a different world back then, and the quality of the milk was undoubtedly better, but it still does not change the laws of chemistry. Mankind's biochemical makeup has essentially not changed. Our *blueprint* still shows us that milk produces these chemical reactions that I described previously, even if it is raw,—straight from the teat.

Two additional developments around dairy products worth mentioning are, again, that several *future trends* companies predict that dairy is in a fade-out position. Vegan alternatives are growing to record numbers and will make the dairy market pretty much collapse by 2030-35. I have already seen the signs that dairy farmers are struggling. Farms are shutting down or being redirected to grow crops, like vegetables, corn, or soybeans. It is challenging to keep up with all the latest developments as things are shifting so rapidly now to improve our lifestyles, but this looks very promising.

There is a western physician committee for responsible medicine representing around 12.000 members that are now urging food administrations to have "breast cancer" warnings on all dairy products. Specifically cheese, because of the reproductive and growth hormones. The *estrogen* in cow's milk increases the risk for various cancers in our bodies, as Dr. C. Campbell's (*China Study*) research found. He even talks about a *trigger* that switches cancer development "on or off" when consuming dairy or when not!

It all makes sense, yes? All the world's mammals have a beautifully designed schedule for the first period of their motherhood. Which is to produce and give raw alive foods in the form of milk to their offspring. And over time, the young one moves on to more solid foods. We are also designed to be weaned off our mother's milk, as healthy and comforting it is. We also need to move on to solid nutritious foods, but by that, I do not mean . . . pepperoni pizza with extra cheese!

With their advertising pitch: "Low fat, eat and lose weight with dairy" the dairy industry has the uninformed consumer easily hooked, but reality draws a different picture. There is a hidden truth that the industry does not want you to know about. It is pretty incredible that they are allowed to use that *loophole* in the food labeling law. It is clearly all about how labels are worded and the industry's economic and political influences. When you check the labeling, you'll see that it is cleverly done. The trick here is to understand the difference between percentage by weight and percentage by calories. Let me draw you an example to show you what I mean:

100 grams of whole dairy contains 60 calories
The weight of 100 grams is broken down like this:

- 88.3 grams of water
- 0.7 grams of ash (solid residues)
- 4.5 grams of carbohydrates
  (x4 calories per gram=18 carb. calories)
- 3.2 grams of protein
  (x4 calories per gram=13 protein calories)
- 3.3 grams of fat
  (x9 calories per gram=30 fat calories

----

100 grams total

Clearly, you see that 88% of the whole dairy product weight is the water, which provides no calories. What is left to calculate is the 3.3 grams of fat out of the total. So, they are putting that on their labels,—3.3% milk fat.

But carbohydrates, protein, and fat do not contain the same energy units or caloric values. Fat has more than twice the amount of calories than carbohydrates or protein, as pointed out before. Each gram of fat needs to be multiplied by nine calories, while the protein and carbohydrates only by four.

So, when we then look at the calories, we see that thirty of the sixty calories in whole milk come from fat. This is where the deliberate confusion is created. You can use this same calculation with so-called low or nonfat milk, ice cream, yogurt, or cheese. This is easy to calculate before you buy.

"But better yet, stay away from dairy all together!"

So, it is clearly evident that we are being deceived. The evil food industry is yet again exploiting another market. They're making money from the biological process of the mother caring for its young. You do realize, by the way, that they take the young calf away within the first 24 hours after birth. Milk flows freely from a nursing mother.

> **On a puzzling side note**—Surprisingly, I once learned that some people think that a cow always gives milk.

Eggs are also counted as a dairy product, even though they do not come from cows, of course. They are unhealthy to eat and are not a chicken's period (*as commonly stated*). Because it is laid by a bird, fertilized or not, it is an animal product that is better not consumed. They have a lot of animal protein, cholesterol, and fat (*about seventy percent*), and you already know the issues around too much protein and fat.

Diabetes—All that saturated fat in an egg can lead to *insulin resistance*. Too much fat, dear reader, is the precursor to an overworked pancreas, not sugar! (*more on page 131*).

Heart Disease—This is a no-brainer. We have to keep our *roads* clear from too much cholesterol (*about 180 mg in an average egg*) and fat so that our blood can be pumped freely.

Cholesterol—Your liver is already producing this essential organic compound, no need to get extra dietary cholesterol. It is just too much for our bodies to handle.

Cancer—Eggs are linked to cancers of the colon, rectal, bladder, breast, ovary, and prostate.

The powerful arm of the egg industry is throwing a lot of unhealthy and untruthful info at you. Please be aware of this.

Dairy, in all its attractive packaging, has become a food item that you will see in almost all supermarket carts. The beliefs in its benefits are deeply rooted, as I brought forward. Free yourself from this lie and find your natural health again! And the next time you walk past a cow or other animal in the field, I suggest to stop for a moment and say,—"Hi!"

When in Transition

If you are that person that needs the idea of milk in your life, then you can make your own from nuts. But I understand that making your own is a job that not everybody has the time or desire for, as easy as it is. In that case, you will find in the health food stores a whole range of better milk choices:

- Almond
- Rice
- Hemp
- Chestnut
- Coconut
- Cashew

The choices are luckily so plentiful that anybody can find an alternative. Pour it over your cereal and fruit dishes, or preferably, drink it as it is. You don't need to miss cow's milk.

Nut milks are incredibly nutritious and generally do not create any problems in your digestive system, as long as you uphold food-combining rules. The safest way is to drink it on its own. Nut milks are great when you need to supply yourself with extra calories, fat, and protein, contained in one single nut and in perfect values. Nut milks (*home-made*), by the way, are the superior alternative to cow's milk when a nursing mother cannot, for whatever reason, breastfeed.

Cheese—And when you found your milk alternative, it is time to face this addiction. Do you know why the majority of people have a hard time letting go of cheese? Well, it interestingly consists of something called "Casomorphins," a casein derived morphine-like compound that acts as an *opiate.* It attaches itself to our brain receptors, like heroin and other narcotics do, so be aware of this. And together with the "Dopamine activity" we have to deal with when eating cheese from cow's milk, we have a tough addiction to battle. Mother nature designed this genius tactic to get the baby cow return to its mother's teats for food, and not for us to get *hooked* on.

And when you liberated yourself from unhealthy cheese, you can find delicious Vegan alternatives in the health food section. Also here there are plenty of choices, so try them out.

Butter—Then we have the many choices of Vegan butter that can get you as loyal to it as regular butter, but at least this time, it will be plant-based goodness.

Yogurt—Still eaten by many as a dessert, sad to say. So try out any of the Vegan ones. Delicious and nutritious.

Ice cream—And last, but not least, we have various Vegan ice creams available in many flavors. When I first had one again after many years, I was blown away! So, if you need to make yourself feel better or console a heart-broken friend, a bucket of Vegan strawberry ice cream will do the trick.

My Cleaner Advice

I used to drink a lot of soy milk, and I loved it. But I stay away now and do not praise them anymore in a clean diet. The convenience of buying prefabricated foods from a store is *unnatural* anyway as foods are designed to be eaten fresh, or at least within the time frame of a few hours.

A Word About Soy

I do not recommend soy products in a clean diet! But before we go into the specifics of why, I need to mention again that soy milks, burgers, and sausages are great transitioning foods for a healthier and guilt-free diet.

The worries and controversies around soy are about the "Phytoestrogens" (*natural plant compounds*), in their most common form called "Isoflavones." They can have estrogenic and/or antiestrogenic consequences and exert their effect on males and females reproductive system. It is called the "Battle of the hormones" as they raise the estrogen levels in both men and women, with possible negative outcomes.

When the estrogen levels in men are increased, testosterone levels will go down, and several effects can follow. Besides an increased waist, a man can find his libido weakened, and the growing of the infamous man-boobs.

When the estrogen levels dramatically go up in a woman's body, possible breast cancer can be created next to irregular periods. Her fertility could also be at risk.

But if soy is truly bad for you or not remains a continuous debate (*thanks to the conflicts between the dairy and soy industry*). When consumed in moderation, I feel that it can be a beneficial transition food. They say that Asians are healthy nations because of soy. But, after a little research, it seems to be the result of marketing propaganda, plus, I personally never see them eat that much soy. (*their lower incidences of heart disease are credited to less red meat and dairy*). Always keep in mind that animal products will do more harm than soy because of their high-fat content. To remind you, make sure that the soy products you buy are from an "organic" source.

I want to leave you with my personal and professional objections about soy, just for you to consider.

These are:

- Soybeans need to be cooked, as straight from nature they are like small hard pebbles, so totally inedible. Indicating clearly that they are not for human consumption.

- The soybean is the number one "Genetically modified" food crop in the world. I am not convinced that it benefits us to modify our food sources to yield better and disease-resistant crops, whatever the food is. Eat organic!

- Tofu, which is eaten by many Vegetarians and Vegans, can be a bit boring. The bland flavor screams for a lot of salt and spices before it is enjoyable, and this is not ideal as you are (*will be*) learning in this book.

- Soy products can produce a lot of gas in an individual, and as we will learn later on, this *rings* trouble. Intestinal conflicts need to be avoided at all times as toxins, created by poor digestion, can become the end product.

- Soy drinks contain processed sugars and are pasteurized, which will *denature* the proteins, kill good bacteria, and destroy active enzymes.

- Soy crops are as harmful to the environment as any other crop when no real smart farming techniques are used. Soils get destroyed with the use of pesticides!

But despite these issues, if you choose to stay Vegetarian or Vegan and so occasionally drink some soy and eat tofu, it will not be that problematic. But when desiring a beautifully clean harmonious system, we follow a *raw alive foods diet*. Then, of course, we stay away from this over-processed bean.

In closing, the best way then for you to drink healthy milk, tricky but possible, is to find a truly raw and unprocessed nut of any kind that you can find in many health food stores. They usually offer our nut family a lot cheaper in bulk or go straight to the importer, as I do. Then, just soak the almonds, cashews, pecans, for a good 24 hours, rinse, and then blend them in a powerful machine with water. Next, pour the mixture through a nut milk bag or cheesecloth (*tea towel can work as well*) and squeeze the liquid from the pulp. You can blend some dates to sweeten the milk with or add fruit for a different flavor, and voilà, you have milk!

If this all feels like too much work, then do what I did. I got myself weaned off drinking any kind of milk. Just get used to drinking freshly made juices or smoothies. They're delicious and nutritious and come summertime crazy refreshing.

Another option, but not often seen as an exciting choice, is to simply drink water. When you have pure and deliciously tasting water, for me, there is nothing better. I am fussy when it comes to water, and luckily I get my water from a well.

Ideally, you avoid buying supermarket water as you never know how long it has been in its toxic plastic container (*generally, I do not drink, but eat my water through fruits*).

Let's explore some other dairy-free clean alternatives:

Yogurt—Raw dairy-free yogurt can be made with raw cashews as they are a creamy nut (*technically, cashews are never raw, just make sure to buy them "unsalted and unroasted"*). A lighter nut-free version can be created with bananas and lemon juice. Add fruit for variety, and some raw date paste as the sweetener (*contact me for the recipe*).

Cheese—And when it comes to cheese, you can make a raw nut or seed cheese. Delicious on a raw cracker or raw flatbread. I personally never liked and ate real cheese (*I am a traitor to my Dutch ancestry*). You can even kinda copy famous cheeses, like *Gouda* or *Camembert*. Find these recipes online and start experimenting. They are soo much more rewarding to consume because you put your own time and love into making it yourself.

Ice cream—And you really do not have to miss out on your ice cream fix for the summertime. Frozen bananas with any type of other fruit, like berries or mango, make a yummy creamy sorbet that is nutritious and healthy. You'll need a kitchen machine or a good household ice cream maker.

Butter—Your savior here is *avocado*. Truly soo much better and healthier. Nice and creamy and perfect for your raw bread. Use sparingly, so the healthy fat will not become an issue. You can also make a raw Vegan pâté to use as butter.

Eggs—As we marked them as a non-food, a lot of people will not be too happy about this. But, for all you "eggivores" out there, we have a plant-based alternative, and soy-free. Just search for: "Vegan egg 'mung bean' recipe."

So, why do we avoid dairy again?

- It is a growth-liquid for baby calves.
- It creates an acid environment.
- It weakens your skeleton frame (*osteoporosis*).
- It contains growth-hormones and other chemicals.
- It contains the wrong problematic lactose sugar.
- It contains too much protein and fat.
- It is pasteurized, and thus unusable (*commercial*)
- It onsets respiratory conditions, like asthma.
- It promotes cancer and diabetes.

I hope you are inspired now to leave dairy behind and commit yourself to explore this new culinary world. Life and food need to be enjoyed! And if you can combine these two, as in, eating deliciously and staying healthy at the same time, I say your mission is completed.

"To eat is a necessity, but to eat intelligently is an art"
- La Rochefoucauld

* * * * * *

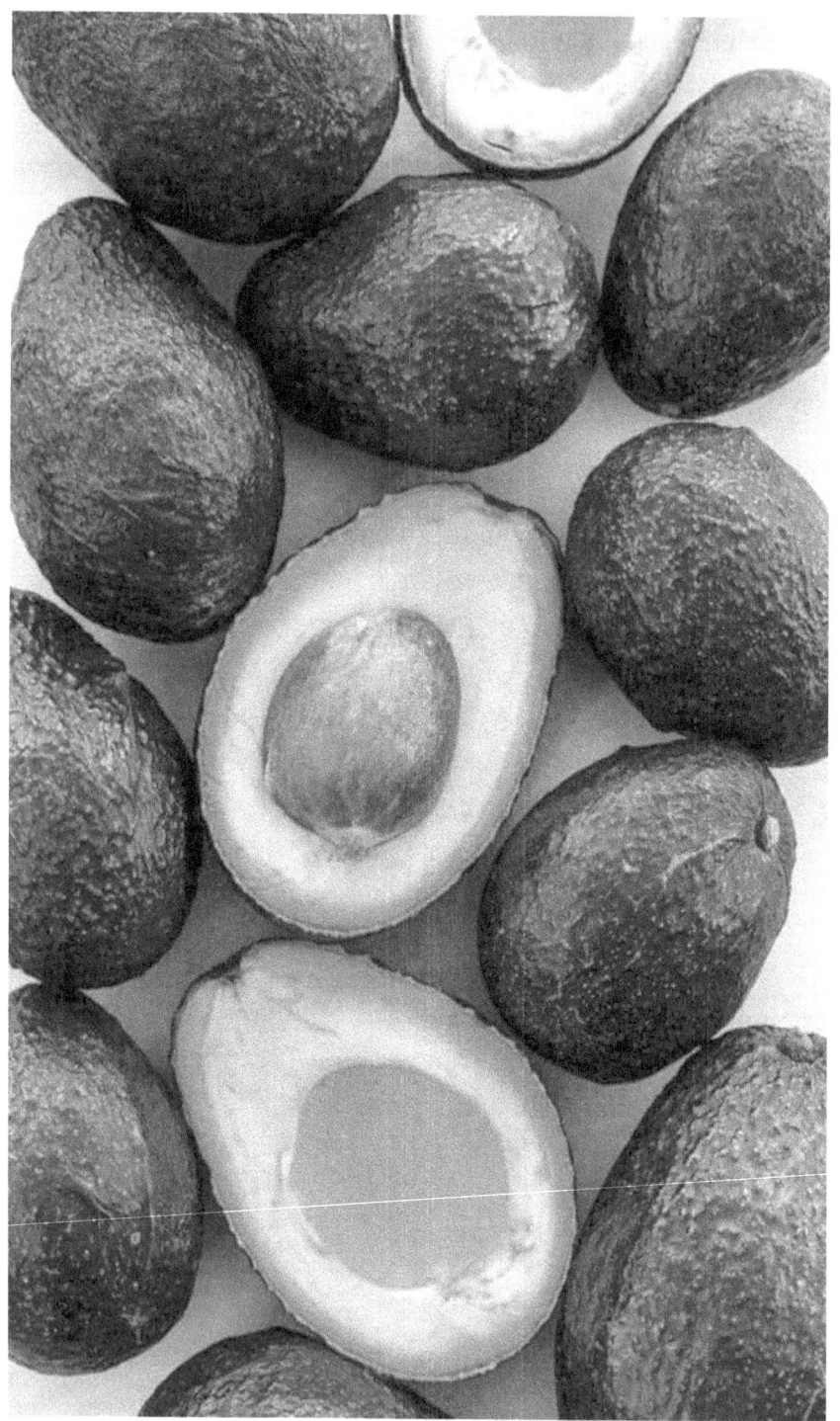

STEP
NUMBER THREE

GRAINS

I can already hear you say: "Oh no, I love my pasta!" And I completely sympathize with you on this one. I used to love spaghetti and macaroni, could eat it every single day. In my backpacking years, and so budget days, that was all I ate because you can buy them everywhere. It is not easy to talk negatively about pasta, bread, and cookies, because most of us grew up with them. We like this food. The times that we stood in the kitchen watching Mom kneading dough, and waiting for the bread or cookies to come out of the oven, are just priceless. And so the problem with this particular *step* is that we will defend the comfort foods made from these grains and thus will deny any good advice that tells us not to eat them anymore. Mostly bread has become, since ancient times, the food of the masses, so you can imagine the difficult task for me at hand here (*first bread was baked around 8000 BC*).

So, for thousands of years, we have been producing flour from grains to make bread. Still, in reality, those millenniums are only a *drop* in the bucket on the scale of human evolution. Thus, cultivating grains is still a very young practice, and ever since those early bread days in history, we have had problems digesting it properly, and we will continue to do so.

Because of ingenious inventions, although primitive at first, we found a way to harvest grains and create flour, which in turn makes bread, pasta, cookies, and many other non-foods. But because we were able to develop these techniques does not mean we should make use of them. Okay, in those days long ago, the bread was indeed healthier than what we currently consume because everything was pure, natural, and free of chemicals. However, it undoubtedly and unknowingly would have created health problems back then as well.

The whole fuss about bread comes from wheat and its problematic ingredient called—gluten. Gluten is that *sticky* molecule that is impossible to be recognized and handled by the body. Besides that, we have a high amount of sugar, salt, and bleached flours in today's manufactured white/brown bread, which is, as you can guess, not very beneficial for your health. As a solution, the health industry has come up with healthier bread in the last several decades, and gluten-free bread is one product of this progress. But still, sorry, bread is a "non-food," an edible sponge. Personally, I feel that it is even a crime to feed it to the pigeons.

I find it indeed a great shame that it is such a problem food. Bread seems like such a great meal, and who can resist that fresh-baked smell? It is easy to carry with you, yummy to smear something on it, and it keeps you good for several hours (*sponge effect*). But I hope that you have learned so far that eating is not a filling-up-your-stomach practice. But that it is all about supplying proper nourishment, and bread isn't going to deliver that to you. Many people's bubbles are burst wide open when they learn about this, and I completely sympathize with the ripple effect it creates.

Increasingly, more consumers cannot eat wheat anymore because of a developed sensitivity to the gluten protein. These individuals suffer from a condition called "celiac disease," which is a genetic *autoimmune* disorder. The diagnostic cases of this condition continue to rise every year. Luckily, good health food stores, as I mentioned, now have many wheat-free options. I tried them once, and some are okay, but the real thing is just way better and makes it so difficult to let go of.

This reaction of the body against the wheat, barley, or rye, by the way, is one to take seriously. I have learned in my studies that everybody reacts to wheat. When the blood is examined after eating a bowl of pasta, for instance, you will discover that the body's white blood cells will start an attack on the elements of the wheat protein (*gluten*). They see it as an "Enemy of the State" (*body*). When they march out, it is not a good sign. The tricky thing here is that not everybody will show immediate symptoms to this sticky invader. This means that many people do not know that the gluten in their diet causes problems and so keep on eating it.

When one organ slowly becomes weakened, it will affect other connected organs, thus, creating an imbalance and poor integrity that will trigger the first bodily symptoms. I worked with a girl once who told me that she got the celiac condition when she was 26, somewhere around her wedding date. She was so puzzled about why she suddenly was suffering for days from these cramps and diarrhea that she was afraid that it could ruin her special day. Fortunately, her well-informed doctor suspected the intolerance to wheat straight away. She stopped eating gluten, and her wedding was saved.

A friend of mine from Spain I visited once started to tell me about her persistent diarrhea, cramps, and bloating issues. When I pointed out that her pantry is filled with wheat cookies, bread, and other non-foods and most likely are causing the problems,—she thought I was mad. Many months later, I get the news that it got soo bad that she went to the doctor. Her physician recommended having a part of her intestines "CUT OUT!" She continued telling me that while she was waiting in the hospital with her mother for this procedure, she suddenly remembered my advice. She felt then that having a piece cut out of her could not be the solution. She canceled and left, stopped eating wheat, and the problem went away. But she has to stay away from wheat for the rest of her life. But no worries, you can live "happily ever after" without wheat because you don't need it. So, these real-life stories reveal an important truth:

"Grains in their raw natural state are for our beautiful birds that have a special digestive system (Gizzard) to handle these tiny seeds with no problem"

They are not designed for human consumption, PERIOD.

It is not fair sometimes is it. I have to clarify that all types of food sensitivities exist these days, even from natural foods. I have met people who could not eat tomatoes, strawberries, or kiwi. Or nuts, like peanuts, almonds, and cashews. The allergic reactions experienced from these nuts can be quite serious, even life-threatening. But these conditions are rare and not entirely the same and do not indicate that these natural delicious foods are not designed for the human race like wheat is. Another reason exists for these food allergies that we, unfortunately, cannot go into here.

If you want to walk the path to radiant health, you will have to let wheat products go. I have come across many amazing articles, real-life stories, and research about wheat that will shock you because of its damage to our health. The fascinating research of "Dr. Kenneth Fine," e.g., reveals the many complications associated with gluten. Positive results were observed with sufferers of "Multiple Sclerosis" that are wheelchair-bound. When the MS diet approach was applied where wheat, eggs, dairy, legumes, and yeast were removed, much improvement in their muscle functions was observed. Also, advancements in the research of "Alzheimer's," a most awful condition, have been observed. It brought intriguing evidence to the light (*but will not see the light of day anytime soon*) that complex carbs, like bread and pasta, are linked to the onset of this dreaded condition as the result of an often irreversible downfall of the pancreas. This alarming situation will starve the brain cells of *glucose*, which it desperately needs! It is more frequently now called "Type 3 diabetes." (*the brain is unable to respond to insulin*). If the importance of the pancreas was truly understood, people would worship it and protect it from harm (*see step seven*).

But these research results are at this time considered very controversial. The agricultural industry is also a huge money-making machine and so heavily defended. It is unthinkable that they would conduct an official investigation on these findings and come forward to state that all wheat products are harmful to people's health. It will just not happen. By the way, these coverups and controversies are also a part of this book as it is crucial to learn about these and not go through life naively. Money still talks, and big companies do not care!

Alternative research that is kept from the public plays an integral part in freeing you of your old reality so that you can live a healthier life. It is simply *not sexy* to have painful cramps, persistent diarrhea, a bloated system,—or worse. The body cannot do its thing when it is obstructed. It wants to keep you healthy, but you will have to do something in return.

"*It is time to make some sacrifices!*"

Also, many people complain about their weight and feel they have tried everything to no avail. You will be amazed when I tell you that as soon as you stop eating wheat, in all its shapes and forms, you will start to lose excess weight. Wheat will blow you up like a balloon. All wheat products will do so because of their irritable unnatural ingredients, salt content (*water retention*), and all other reasons mentioned in this *step*. But no worries, there are alternatives.

I want to share this great questioning *mantra* with you:

> ***"You might love that food, but does that food love you back?"***

Bread is a non-loving food. Leave it alone as it serves you no purpose. It can make you ill,—or even mad!

Many years ago, I read an article, and I loved it ever since. And this article was basically a brief interview with writer and researcher: Guy-Claude Burger, who wrote the book: "Manger Vrai" (*translates into, "Eat Real"*). Many would call him controversial, but a questioning mind is automatically rebellious when he or she goes against the *status quo*.

Can bread, or any other wheat food for that matter, turn us mad? This was the question he asked when he researched wheat. A great question to ask, I always thought. I know it can make you physically sick, but then a person's physical state can be paralleled to his mental state of being. If you look at our planet's psychological health, I feel that something is not quite right there. Increasingly, we seem to distance ourselves and go against our fellow man. We appear to be on edge and are easily irritated. Could bread play a role here? It is apparent to me that the violating of our natural laws is the root cause of many different types of imbalances. The natural law of *cause and effect* seems to definitively apply here.

In his book, he recounts the experiments he conducted on mice,—and his own loving children. His children were the involuntary test subjects that convinced him that there is something up with wheat consumption. He observed that some people seem to be a bit crazy, that it was normal to be a little "off the charts." He conducted his experiments mostly on mice. He felt that psychologically humans and mice have a lot in common. This claimed craziness that he discovered was apparently ever so subtle in humans, but a different story with his mice subjects. This dysfunction of our behaviors he talks about is not immediately noticeable, and it seemed plausible that because of the vast consumption of bread, and other wheat products, this so-called madness is not noticed. He believed firmly, like me, that delicate biochemical processes are easily off-tune. Their sensitive balance becomes quickly challenged when consuming unnatural food elements.

He observed that the caged mice's behavior in two groups was noticeably different if one group of the mice were fed wheat and the other group a wheat-free diet. The mice fed a wheat meal were more aggressive. They were easily startled and clawed at the person trying to pick them up. The other group was found to better tolerate being handled. A picked up mouse would even stay peacefully on his hand while making a *cage* with the other hand's fingers, but it would gently try to push them aside.

Some mice fed the wheat diet even displayed cannibalistic behavior that took this researcher totally by surprise. He then concluded that this clearly coincided with various aggressive behavioral patterns he also observed in people. The increased nervousness seemed to be the controlling behavior in the wheat-fed mice, which was also discovered in humans.

One day he allowed his children to eat for several days as much bread with butter as they desired, which led to further suspicion that wheat is a questionable food source. One of his kids was a girl who was a talented piano player and never failed to play a tune in time. He noticed that the young girl had lost her counting abilities of the notes from the pieces she was playing. His other kid was found to be constantly arguing with his sister and to have more restless nights of sleep. He remembered that his family became turned upside down and that its daily running became quite unbearable.

It is difficult to pinpoint a specific behavior and blame a particular food for the agitation. Because a food item that will imbalance a person's psychological makeup is obviously intertwined with the total diet and so impossible to detect. Plus, if a person's particular diet continues over a long period, a perceived *normality* will be the result.

Bread is highly addictive, and removing this *non-food* from somebody's diet, together with other wheat sources, will need to be done for a more extended period of time. Only then more positive behavioral outcomes can be observed. Anxiety, aggression, depression, inhibition, and overall nervousness result from an unstable biochemical system. Also, a person's predisposition, possibly the outcome of a generation of *poor* diets, can play an essential role in originating an individual's erratic behavior. He went on by stating that eating gluten heightens the symptoms of schizophrenia and other mental disabilities that our populations suffer from. Who knows how many people could be released from our mental institutions if their diets would be adjusted.

I agree that the constant creation of "foreign particles" (*in whatever unnatural chemical form*) in your delicate living system can contribute to the issues he found with bread. But, as with all reactions, we are dealing here with many possible variables. Some are easier noticed in a person than another. Our chemical makeup is intricately sensitive.

To further analyze and prove his theory, he devised a machine that would measure the spasms noticed in the mice. The group of mice fed white bread had body spasms twice that of the regular wheat-free diet group. With all the gluten present, the wheat group was even four times worse than the previous white bread mice group. In our modern agricultural industry over the last several decades, we have *crossbred* many different species of grains. Who knows what dangerous unknown biochemical *mutations* we are dealing with here.

Frustration exists when you have these laboratory results in front of you because removing wheat from our global diets that create these dangerous molecular changes, is presently pretty much impossible. Global health awareness is growing, but educating the masses of this theory will take time.

One more thing, I have started to find news articles where so-called *experts* are warning us that we need to eat gluten for health. Ha! The wheat producers are now afraid of losing market value, and they'll say anything to keep you hooked.

> **"You don't impose a new theory, you wait until its opponents are dead"**
>
> *- Physicist, Max Planck*

When in Transition

If you have decided now to minimize or hopefully completely banish wheat out of your life, then I am happy that you are listening. To find enjoyable alternatives is not a bit difficult as a good health food store is full of options.

Pasta—One of the best wheat-free alternatives to enjoy is brown rice pasta. Also, shirataki noodles are a must to try. Then, we have various macaroni made out of ingredients, like millet, corn (*make sure it is organic*), pea and lentil protein, buckwheat, and quinoa. Also, rice noodles are delicious.

Bread—When it comes to bread, it is also easy peasy. Any decent health food store usually has a *wheat-free* section with cookies, bread, toast, etc. People with wheat sensitivities are on the rise, so a market for these products has been created. Try them all out until you find one that you like.

Alcohol—For all of you who enjoy an alcoholic drink at times, well sorry, but there is a caution with those as well. Beers and most liquors are made of wheat, but luckily, other options exist if you have to drink them. Or stick to wine.

Do not forget that your taste buds have a memory and that you will have to get used to the new flavors and textures of these alternatives. Give it time and keep on remembering why you are saying: "NO" to freshly baked bread. Bring your new-found wheat-free bread to work with a Vegan cheese or pâté. Co-workers will not care. And to really *test* your bravery, bring your new bread, Vegan butter, and veggie burger with you to your in-law's barbecue party (*they will still love you*).

Luckily, celiac disease is an accepted condition these days. Just let people know that you have a sensitivity to wheat, they will understand. And if you feel like really enlightening the situation, you'll let them know that everybody is susceptible to the stuff,—just most of us show no symptoms, . . . yet.

My Cleaner Advice

It is a bit more difficult to bring you a cleaner alternative for bread, cookies, and pasta. There is no natural food really that can replace them because these foods are so utterly unnatural.

Bread—What is exciting is that the *raw food* kitchens of the world have come up with raw substitutes for pretty much all western food items, and this also goes for bread,—kind of. They create *flatbreads* from a mixture of raw ingredients dehydrated in a special machine where the temperature does not go over 40 C or 104 F, so the enzymes stay alive.

Pasta—I let you know before that I loved pasta soo much in my cooked Vegan days. Well guess what, I am making spaghetti now, and macaroni out of zucchini. You have these great *spiralizer* devices that will create a noodle out of any vegetable that allows it. And together with a raw sauce, I am enjoying my pasta again.

Snacks—As for cookies, candies, chips, and other little bites that you used to enjoy as a crunchy snack in your day, or at movie nights, there are many options there too. I make munchies food with dates or any other dried fruit, and Vegan cheese popcorn from cauliflower, for example. Munch on homemade raw granola with pumpkin, sesame, chia, flax, sunflower seeds, and you have a winner. And to suggest an even cleaner option, how about biting in an organic fresh apple, pear, peach, or carrot? We easily forget that these simple delicious foods are the real gifts of the planet. Take these Earthly powerfoods with you to work, or bring on a hike, in case you suffer an attack of the, well,—munchies.

"Let nature be your inspiration"

Please check out my recipe books and videos that I have out to help you with these at: www.youroriginalhealth.com. A whole new tasty culinary world is waiting for you. Enjoy this new dynamic where the foods prepared will actually bring you true health. Please remember that:

"Only from living well,—you can create well-being"

And talking about well-being. I need to briefly talk about the *conditioned* view around cancer. It is definitively one of the most recognized diseases people fear in our modern time, and we still do not seem to have a handle on it,—or do we? Cancer manifests itself in many different types, or "effects" (*cause and effect law*). You still read about the millions being spent on cancer research, together with the multitude of charity and sports events being organized to collect this money for research. It seems to be a hopeless situation.

Most people still have not learned that food and disease have a connection. They still, consciously or unconsciously, indiscriminately eat anything they want with no thought of consequences. Whenever I claim that all types of cancer have the same cause and that it is a *lifestyle* disease, people look at me like I am from another planet. For several decades now, and billions spent on cancer research. The NH philosophy teaches us that we are breaking many *natural laws* and that the disease not only can be prevented but also reversed with a correction in diet (*when caught on time*).

Of course, being ill is never a straightforward situation, but if you think about it more closely, it makes sense to watch what you eat and how you treat your body.

When I mention that it is all a scam and that the cancer industry is a huge moneymaker, I get strange faces there too. The system does not want healthy people! This is a bitter pill to swallow for some. The truth about why all this time and money is being spent to find a cure-all for cancer is to make possibly *billions* more, while a lifestyle change can be the key. "If this is so, how can a young child then have cancer? Because a child cannot possibly have had a poor lifestyle in his/her short lifetime" (*a question I get*). In these cases, NH states that a child will have inherited a genetic weakness of the parent's poor lifestyle (*or a buildup weakness over several generations*), that manifested in a premature imbalance.

One important fact about any type of cancer is that the disease is never an isolated occurrence, like pancreatic or liver cancer, as cancer always exists in the whole body. It becomes manifested in a weakened organ. Therefore, it is not the solution to "ZAP," the isolated tumor growth with deadly "chemoradiation." The whole body itself needs to be restored to a natural balance by removing the toxic buildup!

NH teaches that when a person's cancer is reversed after "chemotherapy," it was the body itself that could restore health again,—NEVER the radiation. An untold truth is that many patients still die after their chemo treatments, and the reason given is always that the cancer was too far advanced.

People are misguided about what a healthy lifestyle entails. So, it will take time before we can come to terms with what our natural diet actually is. We need our governments who financially benefit from the food industry to start informing the public more honestly. But looking at the last few decades of health movements, we are most certainly coming closer.

* * * * * *

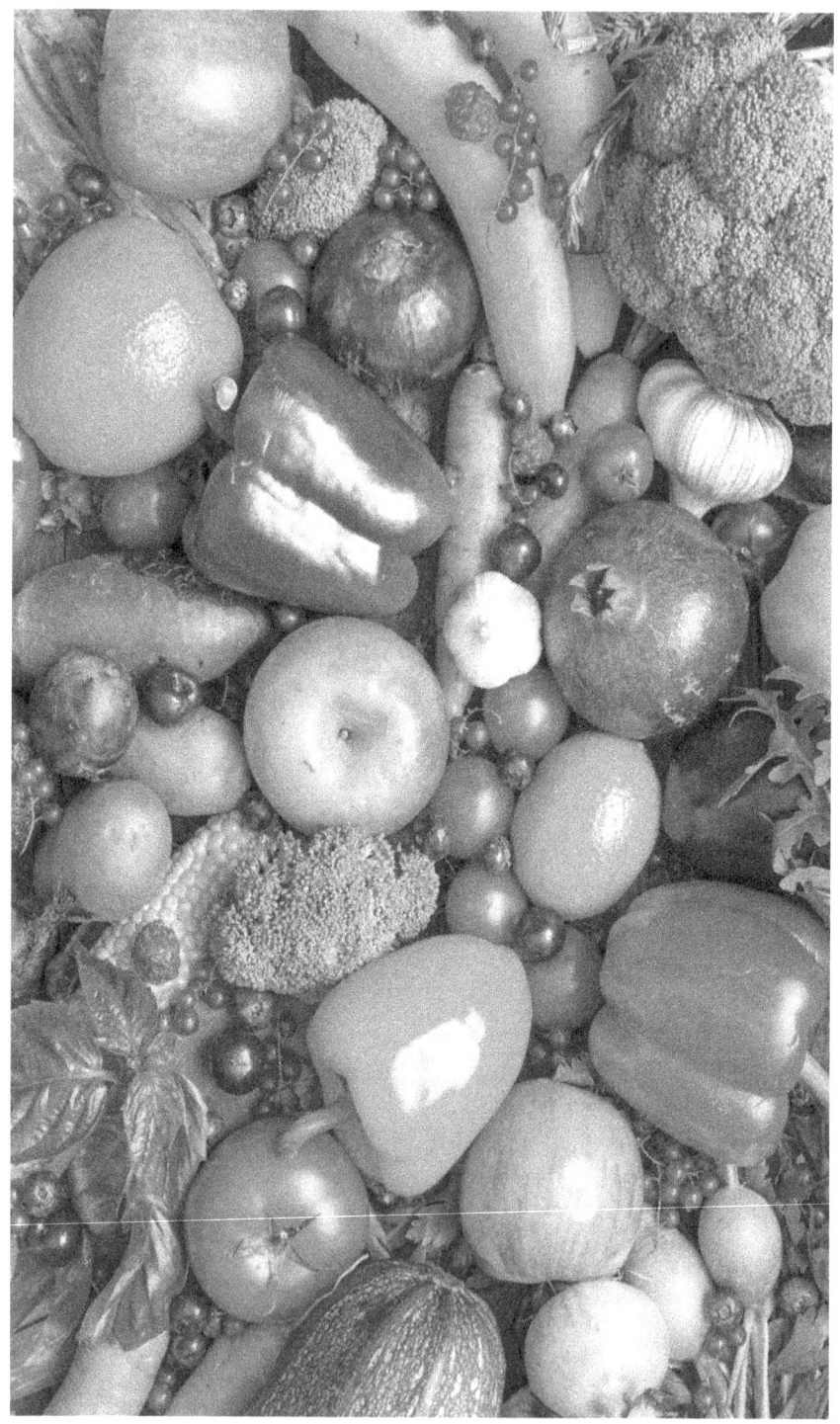

STEP
NUMBER FOUR

FATS

It is estimated by the WHO (*2016*) that around 2 billion adults were *overweight* and of these 650 million were *obese*. These are scary numbers! In today's world of gluttony there are more people dying from body excess than from underweight. Many people do not feel overweight because a lot of folks around them are the same or even heavier. The overall public image of what is considered too heavy is also distorted. Even the standard at the doctor's office and government health branches has changed. We supposed to be much leaner!

Fat is the underlying enemy of our modern-day food intake. More and more, we see children harassing their parents in the supermarket to buy more potato chips and soda pops. With little resistance from them because they are also trapped in the salt, sugar, and fat addiction and are overweight themselves. The image of a person's ideal weight has become warped. Our global health is at risk here, and we need to recognize the enormity of this problem. We are overeating on processed fats, and in my view, we are losing our *dignity* as a species.

Pure unprocessed fat sources can only be found in nature. Fatty fruits, like avocado, coconut, and olives. Also, nuts like almonds, walnuts, and pecans that are technically a fruit have a significant amount of fat. We also have a wide variety of seeds, like flax, chia, sesame, pumpkin, with healthy balanced fat content that is biochemically recognized by the body. These are our fat sources, not, e.g., a plate of "fish and chips."

To many people's surprise, fruits, veggies, and dark greens (*Omega 3's*) also contain low amounts of fats for easy digestion and nutritional density. And together with our fatty fruits and various nuts and seeds, you will supply your body with all the "essential fatty acids" you need.

Side note—All nuts have a high-fat content, and maybe for that reason, Mother Nature housed some of them in a shell that is not easy to crack. A clear sign perhaps to consume sparingly? There is no real scientific evidence for that, but just an observation from your author. Enjoy in moderation!

Any person who observes more closely will see that the world around them is too fat (*people and food*). Eating, as we learned, is an addiction that can be paralleled with a drug dependency. Too often, we see individuals walk around with huge *unhealthy* bodies that can result in social isolation as "fat-shaming" is a real social problem today with often serious consequences. These negative emotions associated with being overweight can bury a person into a dark deep psychological hole that is covered up, layer by layer, by eating more fat for comfort. And to make the situation even worse for an obese person, toxins, and also negativity, are more easily stored in fat, and they are difficult to move when not, well, moving.

For each extra 9.3 calories that enter the body, one gram of fat is stored. That does not seem to be that much, but for every 3500 extra calories, one pound (*0.45 kilos*) is added, and gradually an overweight body is built. And with today's fast-food market, it is very easy to go over your daily caloric requirements and beyond.

We are in trouble here. So, let's sum up the many problems you can encounter when consuming too much fat:

⟩ Blood cells *stick* together, creating less surface area to oxygenate the blood.
⟩ *Obstructs* the delivery from simple sugars to the cells.
⟩ Promotes pancreas *imbalance*, thus, onsetting diabetes.
⟩ Stimulates *overeating*.
⟩ Heating fat will produce dangerous *Maillard molecules*.
⟩ *Stores* toxins and negative emotions more easily.
⟩ Obesity can cause social *isolation* and *depression*.

The food industry has its commercial deceptions regarding fat also lined up for you. Olive oil is surely one of the most famous ones. This oil is praised for its benefits observed in the Mediterranean nations of having low incidences of heart conditions, and I believe this to be partly true. But let's be clear here, heart disease kills many people in those cultures as well. But then these countries cannot really be compared with e.g., the North American population. The Mediterranean diet is just different. It is still more freshly prepared, so less processed on the table. They also still (*thankfully*) live up to their heritage and take their time to eat. So, when a deficient diet is consumed (*eating in a hurry and processed*), don't be tricked in believing that olive oil can come to your rescue.

We cannot fool ourselves by thinking that these oils are good for your heart. How can dietary oil be healthy if it has the potential to seriously block up your arteries? First, oils are too concentrated for consumption, and second, they get used for frying in our western world's poor diets. Two teaspoons of "extra virgin organic cold-pressed oil" of any kind should be the maximum that one takes in daily. And preferably added to the last meal of the day (*more on that in a moment*).

Refined fats are the hidden evils in processed foods, and people are not really informed of the health risks because of dishonest food labeling and adverts. Luckily, when people's awareness grows, manufacturers will adapt. Take "trans fats," for instance. Since 2013, the food regulators declared them "unsafe" for consumption. But although the dangers of trans fats (*partially hydrogenated oils*) are now known, many still consume them in their daily diet. Especially any "deep-fried" foods are a serious health caution! Since the outcry about trans fats in many foods, the American FDA and the European EFSA food regulators recommend these fats to be replaced with "unsaturated" vegetable oils, like canola, soy, or corn. Even though many countries have an enactment in place to limit trans fats use in foods, too much is still consumed.

The issue around fat is not rocket science. It is a clear case of *cause* and *effect* as processed fats clog up your arteries. Clogged arteries cause heart failures, especially if you have a predisposition in your family. There is no real need on my part to convince you that fat is bad. The challenge here is to have you leave it alone. It's essential to have, but only needed in small amounts. So, let's go and see what we can do to minimize its consumption. If you have taken my advice from the first two *steps,* you are already taking charge of your health as you removed a lot of fat from your diet.

When you *overeat* on fat calories, you will *undereat* on carbohydrates. With this, I am informing you that you need to consume a higher amount of carbohydrates. When not eating a sufficient amount of valuable dense nutrients, the body will start asking for more food. A person can be overweight and starving at the same time. Fat fills up a lot quicker than eating fruits, but fat obstructs the delivery of valuable nutrients to the cells. The idea here is to warm you up for the practice of eating more fruits so that you can avoid the temptation of eating fatty foods. But one orange, a pear, or two apples, will not cut it, of course.

Let me list here the fats in our daily foods that
can obstruct your health potential!

- The excessive use of salad dressing or olive oil.
- The use of animal butter on your bread and toast.
- The cooking oil or butter when (still) frying food.
- The consumption of meat, poultry, and fish.
- The consumption of dairy and cheese.
- The consumption of any kind of fast food.
- The excessive consumption of nuts.
- The excessive eating of sweets that convert into fat.
- The indulgence in potato chips and buttered popcorn.
- The overuse of natural fats, like avocado and coconut.

When in Transition

What we are going to do now is to slowly remove the bad fats from your life. Like in the previous *steps*, we will exchange them, food for food, for the healthier and Vegan option. We are also going to opt for foods that are not fried. Then, you look for healthier low-fat munchies in the health food store. It will take some exploring and tasting, but I think this is fun as you are doing this for that new sexy person you will become.

In time you will be automatically more aware of what to buy. Also, if you can, eat a concentrated fatty dinner only every other day (*until your system works more efficiently*). This way, your body will have the opportunity to fully digest the fat before you *download* more fatty foods. Doing this, you also will start to *reset* your system.

In the "Raw food world" it is well-known that the newbies, those who have just switched to this life-giving diet, overeat on fat too. But this overeating of natural fat also happens with veterans who have been eating raw for years, as they are stuck in their belief that as long as it is raw, it is good. A large daily intake of avocados and nuts is normal to them.

Again, the advice here is to limit your intake. So, when you feel the habit coming up of smearing something fatty on your raw cracker or wheat-free bread, is to use a Vegan margarine or spread. They are definitely as delicious as regular butter or cream cheese but a much healthier plant-based choice.

When using a Vegan cheese/spread in a meal, or anything similar, make sure that this dish is prepared with one type of fat. Why one type of fat? Because then you can better control the indulgence of your fat intake, plus, several different fat sources digest with more trouble than just one type of fat. For example, if you take a raw cracker, add a slice of soy cheese and sprinkle olive oil and cut almonds over it, well, that is asking for digestive trouble—and weight gain.

"We need to ascertain that our digestive system is less than burdened, so that we assist it the best we can for a swift digestion"

I do not want to make it too complicated for you here, but I will be happy if you start eliminating the animal fats for now and replace them with your "Vegan alternatives." Ideally, you adapt the routine of eating a fruit meal in the morning and then eating some wheat-free bread or pasta dish with plenty of salad and vegetables for lunch. To then finish your day with maybe a veggie burger gently heated in little coconut oil with plenty of fresh (*always*) vegetables/greens. You will make me proud because it would mean a great new start to a healthier you. It is all possible once you put your mind to it.

One important tip that I want to leave you with is to use coconut butter as your new oil for baking or frying. Coconut is the most resistant oil against heat (*until a certain degree*). Other types of oil turn rancid quickly and transform rapidly into those dangerous molecules we talked about. And anytime you can prepare your food through *steaming* will always be the healthier choice. "Be kind to your food!"

My Cleaner Advice

The strategy when aiming for a cleaner diet is to really limit your fat intake. And the very little fat you do eat will be from a natural, unprocessed source, like avocado, coconut, olives, cocoa, nuts, and seeds. As a reminder, a cleaner menu routine produces fewer food obstacles resulting in the smoother operating of your bodily functions. When you eat cleaner, you will be eating more fruit, vegetables, and greens. They are the fast-digesting alkaline-forming foods (*also containing small amounts of fat*). They are the original foods that we find in our *natural pantry*, stocked by—Mother Nature. And you know that mom always knows best.

When eating more fruit, it is crucial that those simple sugars, vitamins, and nutrients, travel their way through the bloodstream as quickly as possible for a clear passage to your cells. When you drive along a one-way road, you will be forced to hit the brakes when there is another car blocking your way. This is a fat molecule, hindering you from driving your new *electric car* to its destination. These obstacles in the road will create serious traffic jams over time. Make sure that you keep the road clear!

You eat your fat ideally with the last meal of the day and make sure that no sugary foods will be put on top in your stomach (*fruit and desserts*). Your sweet meal can otherwise create a conflict in your gut, producing a foul reeking, toxin forming, over-acidic stomach content (*more on page 140*).

This practice is called "sequential eating." Making sure that the easier digesting foods are eaten first, and the heavier ones come later on. This is crucial when you desire harmonious food digestion, so keep this practice in mind. With no toxins and acid-forming elements roaming inside the body, you can prevent these from diseasing your beautiful you. I want to leave this *step* with some basic guidelines that will prevent you from blaming fruits for any possible stomach conflicts.

SWEET / SUB-ACID / ACID

Fruits fall under specific categories, and they can only belong to any of these above. It is essential for that reason that any fruit you eat combines well with the other. To really keep this rule as simple as possible, when preparing a fruit meal, you make sure that the ingredients are all of the same family, so to speak. Making a yummy dish with sweet bananas? Make sure that the other fruit(s) is/are also a sweet fruit. If you have to stray from that rule (*you can, to some extent*), you then just take a fruit that is next to the other. For instance, you can take a *sweet* fruit and combine it with a *sub-acid* one. What can create a possible digestive challenge is when you combine that same delicious sweet fruit with an *acid* fruit. Also, a *fatty* fruit will only combine well with a sub-acid or acid one, but not very well with yummy sweet fruit. Combine also a sub-acid with an acid fruit.

"Mono-mealing" refers to eating one type of fruit at any given time, so no conflict occurs, and thus the better way to eat fruits. Then what about lunch and dinner combinations, you might ask. All vegetables and salad greens combine pretty well with all fruits. When you eat something heavier, like a veggie burger, you would have to technically eat the fruit first, wait 30 min, and then eat the burger. But nobody really does that. So, just eat fruit separate from main meals or only after, or with, a veggie/salad meal. These are simplified rules, try it out, and learn from what your body is telling you.

Below you find a short NH list to give you an idea to where your new friends belong. Enjoy them!

SWEET	SUB-ACID	ACID
• Bananas	• Mangoes	• Oranges
• Cherries	• Berries	• Pineapples
• Persimmons	• Apples	• Kiwis
• Cherimoyas	• Peaches	• Strawberries
• Fresh and dried figs	• Pears	• Tomatoes
• Fresh and dried dates	• Plums	• Lemons
• Grapes and raisins	• Apricots	• Cranberries

* * * * * *

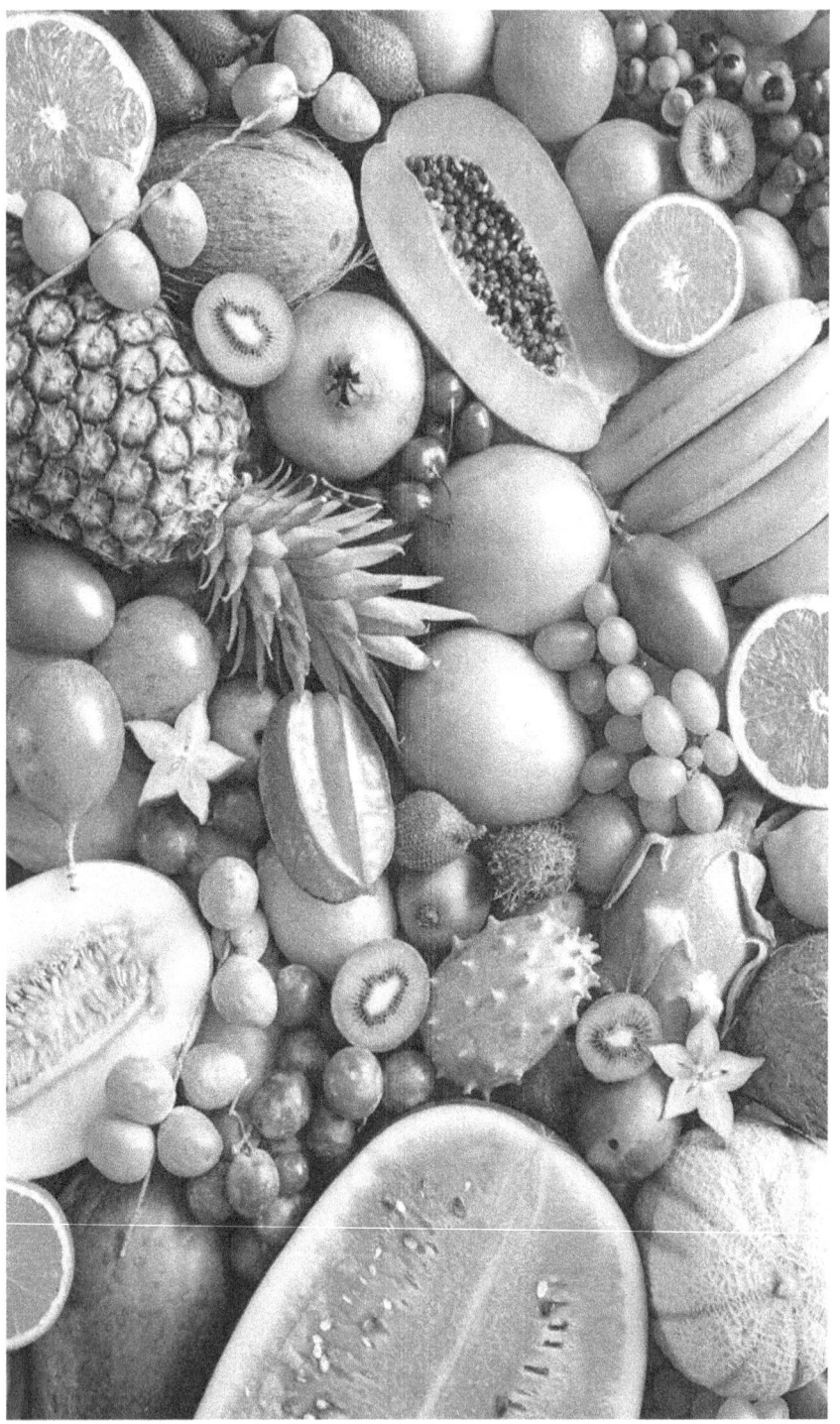

STEP
NUMBER FIVE

SALT

We face a well-known adversary here, so let's put it on the table and scrutinize its properties. And usually, our subject is literally on the table in the form of table salt. Like fat, the average consumer these days is well aware of the dangers of salt. The elderly are often advised by their doctor to lower or halt their salt intake, as the risk for creating high blood pressure, so heart attacks, increases with age.

Let's start by stating that salt is a "Protoplasmic poison." And therefore, it creates various imbalances in your cell structure. But let me first lift the veil on the confusion that exists when it comes to the consumption of salt. Most people know that we need salt to survive. Indeed, we need salt for:

- Cell functioning
- Brain health
- Kidneys
- Liver
- Blood
- Metabolism
- Fluid balancing
- Libido (*male / female*)

But the fact is that we need "sodium," which is an essential mineral/nutrient occurring in natural food, and not the "salt" (*sodium and salt are not the same*) that you find in little bottles on restaurant tables. Also, all the Frankenstein (*dead*) foods contain salt. Sodium can be found more abundantly in dark greens, like spinach, kale, chard, celery. This mineral sodium is chemically recognized by the body and then fully utilized. It also helps to restore your natural taste buds again.

Health problems associated with the overuse of salt, but also with a deficiency in natural sodium, are numerous, and these are largely ignored by mainstream media. Moreover, their names are used interchangeably. We also have been told that salt *retains* water, but this assumption is not entirely correct. What table salt actually does is to encourage the body to use its water to dilute the bodily fluids, so that the toxic properties of salt have less effect on the system. We can rely on this intelligent protective action only to some level though.

> **"When you push the boundaries of any action it will eventually fail on you"**

It is quickly proven that table salt or "sodium chloride" (*40% sodium and 60% chloride*) is an irritant that needs to be shielded from the delicate tissues when one sprinkles salt in an open wound or eye. Very sensitive nerve endings along your whole digestive track become quickly desensitized by the body's defenses against this, or any other, poisonous element. Salt is added in high amounts to pretty much all processed foods, so its acceptable daily levels are easily exceeded. Therefore, to control healthy sodium intake, you consume it only through natural foods.

When a body is constantly being enervated by exposing it to any type of irritant, the body's defenses become weakened, and the essential functions for body integrity will go down. When a fully energized and clean body is exposed to too much table salt, it will immediately respond by removing it through vomiting or diarrhea. So, it is crucial that those defenses stay alert and fine-tuned for your protection.

If you find yourself stranded on a deserted island or in a lifeboat floating on the Pacific Ocean, you would be tortured by the reality that although you have all the water around you that you need, you cannot drink it. Drinking saltwater would dehydrate you even faster in the hot sun, and you will die shortly if no fresh water at hand.

A side note—It is just unbelievable the health scams they come up with these days! Like, *bottled seawater* from great depth where supposedly the ocean is not polluted, and so more nutrient and mineral-rich for better hydration (?)

Another indicator of salt's toxic abilities is when you give salty water to a flower, a seed, or a tomato plant. We all know what will happen (*the exceptions are the marine plants and other species adapted to thrive in saltwater*). Remember that you are connected to your outer environment. Your inner environment exists on the same principles, the same natural laws. Thus, processed salts destroy your natural equilibrium. So, when eating those salty dead foods, you will unavoidably dehydrate and poison yourself. To continue is a path to self-destruction and early aging (*to put it dramatically*).

When consuming a *natural sodium* diet, as I recommend, you rarely need to hydrate with water (*only when exercising or hiking*). As you will be, besides eating your water through a high fruit/veggie diet, avoiding an imbalance in your cells that you would otherwise have to correct by drinking water. If you finished a meal and are later on plagued with intense thirst, you have created that imbalance in your cells. You have taken in too much salt and/or spices.

Salt is a tricky element, as our bodies continuously crave it. When consumed in an unnatural and toxic property, the body starts to form a liking to it, which turns into a dependency. When a person eliminates the toxic salt from their diet, the body can actually start to crave more salt, as a last cry before it is freed from it. This is understandably so, because the body then is seriously deprived of usable salt minerals, so it is screaming for the real thing. Each and every single cell of all your "trillions" of cells (*billions more or less depends on body size*) has its cellular integrity threatened when consuming this poison. When this happens, your inner-cell structure will change for the worst. The essential "potassium" mineral in the cell will soon be lost in the urine, creating further imbalances. Tissues that have absorbed the salty diluted body fluids will lose their elasticity and begin to constrict.

Potassium—I need to emphasize here the importance of sufficient potassium levels in your system. Potassium and salt are connected, meaning, when your salt levels rise, potassium levels go down. It is an important "electrolyte" that regulates many essential functions. A low potassium level can result in insufficient insulin production that can lead to high blood sugar, making you a possible candidate for diabetes. Keep your healthy levels up through our natural foods, like bananas, avocados, and tomatoes. Watch excessive depletion through sports by sweating or by frequent urination.

The continuous high salt intake with the loss of valuable potassium will cause the muscles, valves, and the arteries to shrink and calcify, which will trigger to destroy your tissue equilibrium. Salt can cause a depletion in *collagen* and will draw out water from your skin, resulting in early wrinkles and "unsexy flabby skin." Drinking/eating sufficient water, plant foods, and natural hydrating skincare are your best defense!

"There is no faster way to look and grow old with all sorts of ill conditions than to keep on riding the salt train"

And "on-board" as well is the overconsumption of alcohol, chemical drugs, and smoking. So, I hope I have convinced you now to eliminate toxic table salt from your life and to increase your *natural sodium* levels. Take your time to wean yourself off it. Never forget that your instincts and taste buds have become corrupted. Luckily, they can be restored to their full glory so that you can start to taste real food flavors again.

When in Transition

The wise decision to lessen and ultimately remove your table salt intake is better made in steps. Do what I did many years ago. Add just a little less than the last time when adding salt to your food. Remember that your body will start to crave it more intensely when cutting yourself free too abruptly. Look for foods that contain quality sea salt, which is ALSO toxic, unfortunately, but a lesser evil when transitioning. Keep on checking the salt content labels and when food has more than 1 gram of salt on 100 grams of weight, leave it!

Even Vegetarian and Vegan health foods contain salt, don't be fooled into thinking that they don't. Also here there is no real other transitional option than sea/rock salt (*non-iodized*) with no chemical additives, and to watch the amount you use.

See yourself as training for a big competition, be strict with yourself. Know why you are in this *race*, what it will take to win, and what your victorious reward will be in the end. And don't forget to congratulate yourself occasionally.

My Cleaner Advice

Of course, total abstinence from salt is your new road, and a diet high in sodium your light at the end of the tunnel. A high *natural sodium* content food that needs to be recommended here as the very best source is—vibrant green celery. Not everybody is a fan of it, but it contains high levels and is perfect for supplying the body with this essential mineral. If you do not like the intense taste of celery, you can juice it (*eating it whole is still better*) with some carrot and/or apple. It is a great alkalizing drink/food to start the day with. These green sources of sodium are indeed—"superfoods."

A possible challenge to all parents is that kids (*some adults too*) are known to "kick and scream" at the sight of green food on the table. So parents, stand your ground.

All our fruits and various nuts and seeds have also trace amounts of sodium under their skin. When a variety of these is consumed, you will provide the body with all you need. A renewed trust in our natural foods needs to be built if we want to succeed in health and rebalance what is lost.

Another concern that needs to be addressed is the "iodine" issue, as you need to be informed that it is essential for our thyroid. Salts are *iodized* and are one source for people for this mineral, besides dairy products and eggs. But to promote salt consumption for this mineral is absurd. Another source involves eating our creatures of the sea. Luckily, healthier animal-friendly ways exist. How about bananas, strawberries, cranberries, prunes, zucchini, broccoli, and cauliflower, (*levels depend on soil*) and dried sea vegetables, like seaweed.

I also need to mention the many varieties of condiments that enhance cooked food's *bland* flavor and have become an addiction. These flavor enhancers are considered toxic in the world of "Natural Hygiene" because they are, after all, not a wholefood and will irritate the cells on contact. Spicy peppers especially will irritate your delicate membranes (*try to rub some in your eye*). The mucus the body produces is essential for different body functions, lubrication, protecting organs, and it collects bacteria and irritants. Extra mucus is produced when it needs to protect you from the harm that is being done. We all have experienced, besides when having a cold, a runny nose after consuming any of these spicy irritants, no? The body flushes these unwelcome guests out the door to maintain its health equilibrium. So try to minimize these seasonings, especially the black, white, and spicy peppers.

The habit of adding salt and spices to your food also contributes to the many dry scalp issues people are battling with. The commercial world tells us that the solution to this itching problem is a chemical anti-dandruff shampoo, but these products are very aggressive to your delicate skin and hair. I tell people that I would not even wash my car with that stuff, which gives them a clear idea of my opinion.

A Restaurant Secret—(*connected to the endorphins discussed on page 28*). All the restaurants in the world, be it Thai, Japanese, Indian, or Spanish cuisine, are all in the business of only one thing, to keep you *hooked* on their food! How? All these foods contain "Three" essentials that the body needs: *fat*, *salt*, and *sugar*. But they exist on menus in the wrong form resulting in the body endlessly asking for the real thing. Yet, these foods still create pleasure. And this is the food addiction that we all face every day. "Exhausting!"

The cleaner and more natural you eat, the more you will not crave salty foods or condiments anymore. It will restore your taste buds and even your eating signals that will let you know what to eat, when your body needs it, and when you had enough,—beautiful really.

* * * * * *

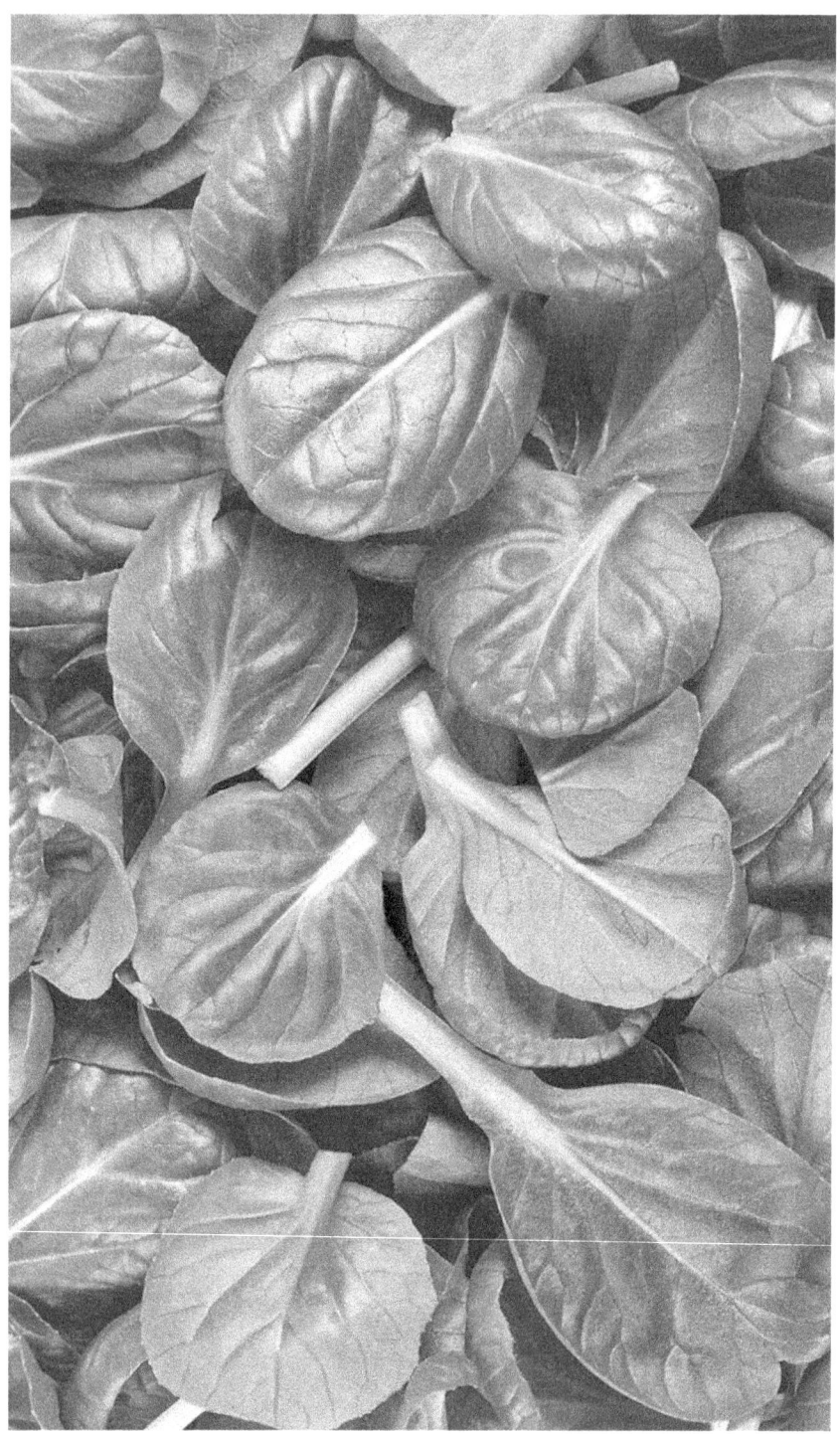

STEP
NUMBER SIX

COFFEE

Ahhh, this should be interesting. So, let's sit down and have ourselves a wee chat about coffee. And I will begin this *step* by listing the possible consequences when consuming this dark bitter liquid. For all of you habitual drinkers out there, it will most certainly burst your coffee bubble,—I sure hope so. For those who wanna skip this "wake up call" (*as you don't feel ready yet to hear this*), I say: "All my respect to you, but you know that it is time to get real with your vices. To face the truth that this addictive brew is not a healthy beverage."

Hold on to your seats, here we go:

- Periodic headaches
- Dwindling energy levels, more fatigue
- Moodiness that can result in depression
- Gastrointestinal imbalances, diarrhea, cramps
- Insomnia
- Irritability, plus panic and anger eruptions
- Constipation, poor bowel movements
- Anxiety
- Involuntary muscles spasm's and pains
- Irregular heartbeat
- Feeling drained all the time
- Lightheadedness
- Stiffness of the joints
- Erectile dysfunction

- High blood pressure
- Ulcers
- Anemia
- Shaky hands
- Ear ringing
- Memory loss
- For woman: Premenstrual symptoms
    Irregularity
    Painful breasts
    Emotional imbalances

Do I need to go on? It is shocking, right? Occasionally, I come across articles that still claim the many health benefits of coffee! The money that is still poured into this commercial propaganda machine is tremendous, please be aware of that fact. You are being conditioned to believe that a few cups a day are actually good for you, so:

"Wake up and smell the—Truth!"

And when you finally decide to kick the habit of drinking coffee, you may have to undergo (*depending on your level of addiction*) unpleasant withdrawal symptoms. But you will come out of those annoyances a new person. And providing you've already started to implement all of your newly learned diet truths, that new person in you will begin to experience the feeling of being naturally energized. Imagine waking up fresh and staying on a high energy trip all throughout the day (*providing you had a good deep sleep*). But to stop coffee and continue eating junk food isn't going to do it, of course.

Before you can experience this "natural energy high" these are the symptoms that you might have to go through:

- ⇨ Some more headaches
- ⇨ Irritability
- ⇨ Muscle issues
- ⇨ Nausea
- ⇨ Memory loss
- ⇨ Intense fatigue

The body has to go through these bothersome withdrawals, unfortunately. But it will be patiently resetting its natural rhythms and functions that will start to give you back that energy, that *original* high, on a continuous level. It will be like hitting a "reset button."

A great book that came out in 2008 called "Caffeine Blues" by Stephen Cherniske, revealed the many problems associated with caffeine. He spent years researching "America's number one drug." But the whole world is addicted to coffee, and people from all walks of life cannot start their day without it. It is a touchy subject as we will always defend our drugs, especially when it is experienced beneficial and harmless.

There are obvious reasons why people drink coffee. I have observed this numerous times in hotel lobbies where you can find these big coffee machines brewing all throughout the day. I would watch the hotel guests walking around with their big mugs filled up to the brim. That routine is, of course, not only privileged to hotel residents but at home as well. "We have to drink coffee to make it through the day!" It becomes the unceasing routine to not let yourself feel the caffeine low by drinking more before it hits you.

And why do people drink coffee? For—energy. The belief that it will bring you an energy boost is truly a misconception that is blindly believed and experienced by many drinkers. The caffeine will indeed provide you with an extra *boost* that is perceived as an increase in physical/mental energy. But, in fact, it is a reaction to the toxic properties. The caffeine will rob you of your precious natural energy that your body stores for many functions. And like anything that is taken, at some point it will need to be claimed back!

Important News Break—NO known substance in this world can give you more energy! There is nothing in a pill, drink, natural food, or physical activity that produces more energy (*sports kick-start your energy, but does not create more*). You have a set amount of energy levels that are always at your disposal. You just have to utilize these levels properly according to the "Laws of Excitation." Herbert Shelton, the father of *natural hygiene*, states:

"Whenever any irritating substance or influence is brought to bear upon the living organism, this occasions vital resistance and excitation manifested by increased and impaired action. Which always necessarily diminishes the power of action, and does so in precisely the degree to which it accelerates action. The increased action is caused by the extra expenditure of vital power called out, not supplied, by the compulsory process, and therefore the available supply of power is diminished by this amount. Under all circumstances, vitality or energy of any character whatever is invariably manifested or noticed by us as energy in its expenditure, never in its accumulation."

In other words, what appears to give us energy is actually draining our precious energies. The stimulation people get from drinking coffee, or any other caffeinated source, is an expenditure of crucial vital forces, not the creation of valuable energy. You have a set amount of natural energy storage, and when depleted, it needs to be restored. That can only come from a deep healthy sleep, as I explained. Let me take this a little bit further. There is only one real source of energy: your "vital" or "life-energy," created in your beautiful brain. The recharging of your lifeforce can only happen during your daily practice of sleeping. There is no other way! We all know that when we are tired and go to sleep, we will wake up feeling refreshed and ready to take on another day. But the misunderstanding happens when we think that if the night of sleeping, for whatever reason, did not produce enough energy, we can add or create some more by artificial means.

Most people, if not everybody, have experienced this at least several times in their lives through whatever stimulant. The illusion of feeling energized through product "X," and then to only crash at the end. I have personally observed the dangerous side effects of the drug "Ecstasy." Where its users can dance all throughout the night until the early mornings on top of a whole day. To then crash and fall into a coma sleep for 20 hours or more to recover. It really is like "catching up" on sleep and restoring your energy reserves that have been seriously depleted by ignoring natural laws.

So, the secret to feeling energized early in the morning and throughout the day is to prevent unnecessary *enervation* to the body. To make sure that your levels never go down too much. You need to make sure that the body has plenty of reserves left for the job of operating the important bodily functions. We learned that one of the key tasks is removing an excess of toxins that otherwise inevitably leads to—toxemia.

Another interesting observed consequence is that coffee is responsible for a lot of miserable people on this globe. The irritable mood swings, often associated with coffee drinking, are greatly underestimated. Oh my, do we ever get *cranky* in the morning if we do not get our fix. It is not the natural way to be. You will become stuck in a perpetual state of false energy and fake uplifted spirits, to then crash and become fatigued and moody. It is extremely exhausting, you have to admit. This chemical stimulation is actually the body dealing with increased stress hormones. In reality, it is deceptive alertness, as there are no real observed improved motor and mental functions when *infusing* yourself with this drug.

Some people seem to tolerate it pretty well (*so they think*). Possibly, they are not as affected as everybody else as we all have a different toxin removal setup (*meaning good or poor, old or young*). The more your body takes in poison and adapts to it, the less resistant it becomes, and the more poorly the body expels it. Look at children that consume coffee for the first time (*kids react in disgust when drinking it*). They can literally fly off the roof after their first few sips. It clearly shows the instant poisonous effect this dark liquid has when consumed on a pure clean system, like that of a child.

Please forget about that moderation message that one cup a day is healthy for you that you find in the media. It is not true. We are conditioned to believe it, and we look for excuses to accept it. These are all signs of denial and, unfortunately, reflect the behavior of a drug addict,—if you like it or not.

I learned that coffee was initially used as a medicine. There was a point in history where toxins were administered to patients because it was believed it would heal them. In a way, this procedure is still around as many medications contain caffeine as their active ingredient. But the trouble really started when a long time ago, monks discovered that you could roast these toxic beans and make a drink out of it. Soon after they discovered that people stayed awake a lot longer, a new *miracle* drink was born. For cultural traditions, it came in handy. For instance, when there were long religious masses held, you would not fall asleep during prayer. When it was introduced to Europe by early explores, it was received as a most repellent drink, but when the addictive energizing qualities were discovered, people started to make an effort to find a way to make it palatable,—sugar. The new beverage was hailed as a tremendous discovery and an addition to the rich cultures of Europe.

It is interesting to know that we have always been looking for ways to "disconnect" ourselves from the burden of reality. Occasionally, we discover a new *escape route*, but presently we are being drugged by alcohol, coffee, cigarettes, (*I am including "vaping" here, which now turns out to create fatal lung conditions, due to its added chemicals, especially, "Vitamin E Acetate"*), marijuana, and energy drinks, as well as potent drugs, like heroin, cocaine, and pharmaceuticals. Of course, any of these have varying degrees of addiction effect, but they all still fall under the umbrella of escape substances, an exit from daily life for the body and/or mind.

I need to also mention the "hallucinogenic" substances that we use to explore our subconscious with (*despite still being illegal, they are coming out of the dark, and its benefits slowly recognized*). The natural ones (*psilocybin mushrooms, ayahuasca, DMT, mescaline*) have deep Shamanic roots because they come from Mother Nature herself and have been around since the beginning. Personally, I feel that they cannot be placed, like man-made drugs, under that umbrella. These mysterious natural grown compounds have a very profound purpose in our lives, yet to be discovered by many.

To me, it is clear why people wanna run away from their reality. It is obvious why we choose to change, suppress, or enhance our realities with various drugs because we can feel trapped. We are often depressed and unhappy as we are living in a challenging, stressful world.

It is much more rewarding to "thrive" on natural energy. It is after all, besides life itself, the most valuable gift from Mother Nature. Our natural energy and health are seriously threatened by what coffee does to us and what it actually contains. For starters, it is made of various unsafe acids, like "Methyluric acid" that tallies heavily to the body's acid burden. In its natural state, caffeine is actually a biological poison acting as a pesticide. It paralyzes and kills insects that attempt to feed on the plants. (*ah, the intelligence of the natural world*). Furthermore, the beans contain several dangerous chemicals, most importantly, "Polycyclic Aromatic Hydrocarbon," which is a highly toxic carcinogen and created through roasting. You might remember that dangerous boy as a cancer-causing agent in barbecued meat.

The last thing I would like to mention again is its effect on our sleep patterns, as this can be detrimental to our precious well-being. Natural deep REM sleep is of utmost importance for health. Coffee disrupts deep sleep, which will inevitably lead to an energy shortage, which will then create a buildup of toxins and an oncoming of disease. People express that the drinking of coffee before the evening does not affect their sleep in any way. I doubt this to be true. First, you do not know if they are truthful (*they are defending their drug*), and secondly, maybe to them, a few hours sleep with twists and turns appears like a normal sleep pattern. The dangers of coffee/caffeine are evident when I observe a person in the morning trying to "wake up" by drinking it. Whenever you drink it, it is always a drainer of energy.

I hope I succeeded in helping you out of the *coffee pit*. I know what it is like. I gave it up myself one beautiful sunny Bermuda day in 1995. I remember what it did to me. I started to drink green tea after my coffee habit in my early Vegan days because the cooked Vegan diet also requires a lot of digestive energy. I felt sleepy a lot, and I needed to keep myself *boosted* in my busy life. I understand that you think that you need it, but this need has many consequences for your health in the present and future. One needs to only *shift* one's thought about it.

Please realize that if you are a drinker of coffee or any other caffeinated beverage, . . . it is time to let it go.

When in Transition

The advice I had for you concerning salt can help you with coffee too,—baby steps. Whatever your routine is, start to minimize the amount of coffee that you drink daily. When eliminated too soon, you will undoubtedly feel the after-effects hitting you hard. You can also try for a while to switch to green teas, but be careful not to replace coffee with the same amounts of tea. I mention green teas because I feel that they are the healthiest alternative, preferably an organic one.

Maybe I am asking too much of you now to completely eliminate caffeine from your life. But if you can leave out the coffee, energy drinks, and anything chocolate (*sorry, but has caffeine too*) and stick to drinking only organic green tea at times, you will already be doing yourself a huge favor.

There are great coffee substitutes that can be found in your local health food store. They are made from grains and roots and can have a roasted scent and taste to them, and could temporally or permanently replace your original toxic brew. Caffeine is extremely addictive and energy-draining, so make a real effort to expel it from your life.

My Cleaner Advice

For all of you cleaner bodies out there, I can only advise you to take it a step further. Hot beverages are a risk to your health as the boiling of the water destroys its structure (*wait for my water step*). Besides that, when not careful when drinking, the unnatural hot liquid can slowly weaken and damage the delicate cells of the esophagus, which you do not wanna do. Also, those *fake* coffee's are not whole living foods.

For the sake of drinking something, I can only suggest, of course, to replace all your beverages with fruit drinks, and I am talking about the ones you can make at home, not store-bought. Only when you make something yourself, you will know what is in it. The beauty of fruit is that it doesn't matter if you eat or drink it, you will be getting the valuable water content you need. A juice, smoothie, or fruit meal is truly the best way to start the morning with. Remember that you have been detoxing all throughout the night.

While taking in fruits, you will be simultaneously cleansing your body, as fruit has a high water content and is soo easy to digest. If your first heavier meal is around lunchtime, you will have given your system a sufficient amount of time to pass your morning meal. Your energy levels will be charged and ready to do some more heavy lifting, so to speak.

The water from fruit will help to flush toxins from your body. A more thorough daily "house cleaning" has never been better. (*more tips on our important hydrating will follow when the interesting topic of water is discussed further on in the book*). Try out different juices to make it as tasty and variable as possible. Make sure that you will look forward every morning to your first meal of the day (*drinking juices or smoothies is still considered eating*).

Tip—For all of you waking up in colder climates where a hot drink is often a must. I suggest to heat up a mug and add warm homemade nut-milk (*don't boil it!*). You could add a chocolate substitute called *Carob* (*very nutritious and no caffeine*). Holding an oven-heated mug in your hands and drinking something warm will help in the mental satisfaction.

As we talked about juices and smoothies that you will be making now routinely in your new lifestyle, it will be a great help to have the right tools. A regular kitchen has pots and pans, and in this new culinary world you are about to enter, you will need a powerful blender (*also to make nut milk, sauces, and creams*), and a SLOW-juicer (*this type of juicer does not centrifuge your foods, but instead grinds them up slowly, so the juice stays "raw" and nutritious*).

> **"We are given the gift of life, and it is up to us to give ourselves the gift of living well"**
> — *Voltaire*

* * * * * *

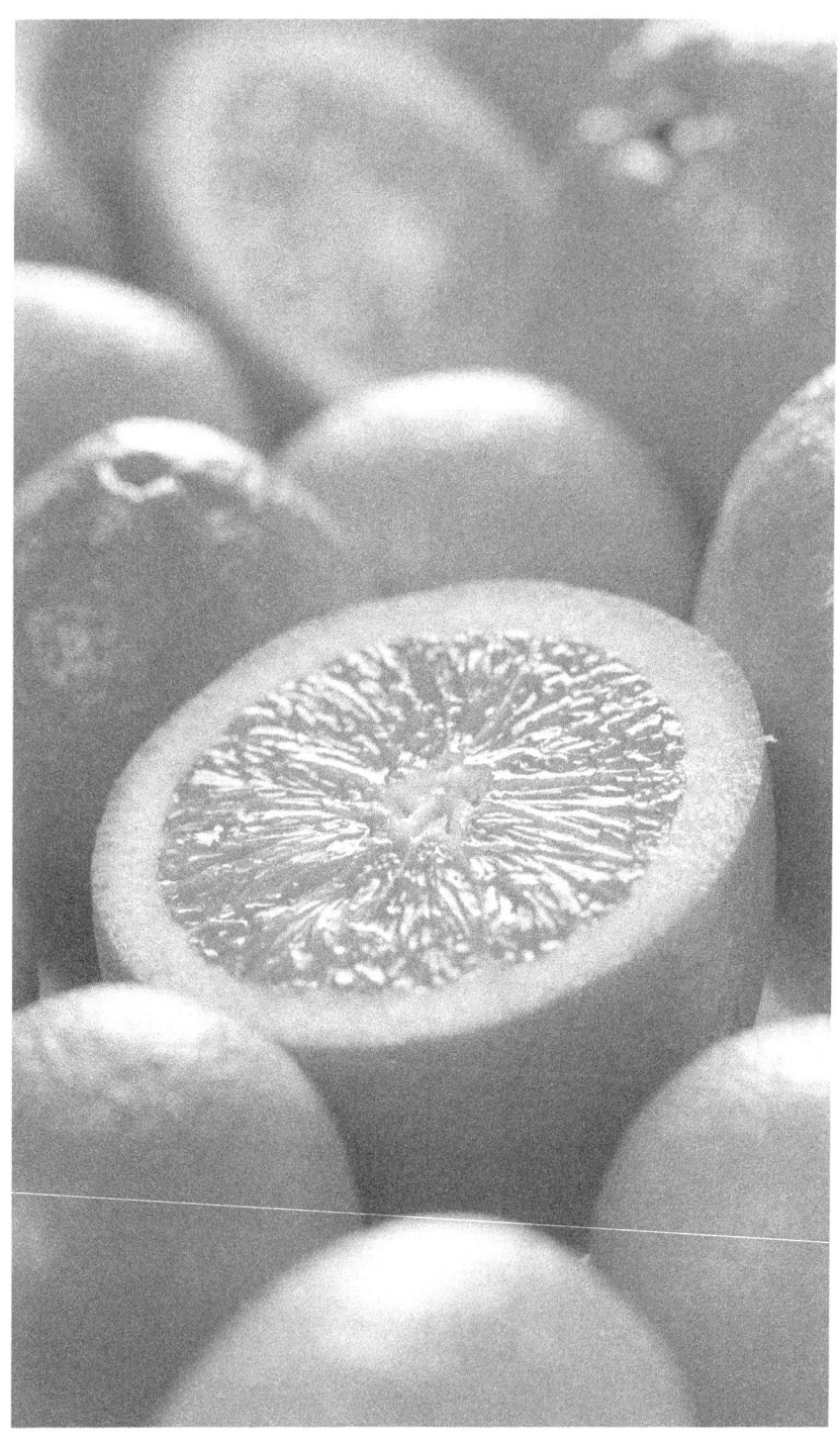

STEP
NUMBER SEVEN

SUGAR

Sugar, . . sweet, sweet sugar. We all have to admit that we are addicted to sugar,—and rightfully so. We are consciously, or subconsciously, looking for this drug every day, and have different sources and suppliers. We consume it at home and in public, and some feel that they need to hide their dependency. Many people are unaware of any addiction and go about their daily lives consuming it with no guilty thoughts. Others, who are aware and scared of sugars fattening abilities, will monitor its intake and try reluctantly to minimize its consumption, but often to no avail. It sure is an exhausting love affair.

Sugar has become a problem for us, a big question mark, as we are struggling with sugar consumption. We do not know what and who to believe anymore in this world of conflicting theories. What are the sources safe to eat? How much can you eat? And is it really making us fat? Too much false info is flying around, and it is time for it to land.

Since the early days of the modern food industry, the *food producers* have been adding this addictive goody to all their processed foods to keep us hooked (e.g., *glucose, sucrose, fructose*). This undoubtedly is no surprise to you. Then, our alerted health organizations demanded stricter regulations because the statistics of increasing obesity were being paralleled to the high sugar levels in food. The food industry complied unwillingly! But with the smart creation of artificial sugars without calories, they found a way to lure customers back to their addicting foods with a NO weight-gain promise. They began to hide these chemical sugars in your food under different names like:

- Saccharin
- Cyclamate
- Aspartame
- Sucralose
- Advantame
- Neotame

These sweeteners are all designed to fool you into thinking that you can still have sugar without gaining weight as they are processed and created in a lab. True, you will not gain weight from these low-calorie sweeteners directly, but the ripple effect they create will surely bring declining health with obesity lingering on the horizon. They even increase the cravings for sweets and stimulate appetite in the brain.

The controversy surrounding these man-made sweeteners continues because of the severe health risks attached to them. Namely, "Aspartame" has been the target (*NutraSweet and Equal*). Adding these sugars to our foods and drinks, together with the confusing and promotive "low sugar, lose weight" labels, guarantees our unceasing addiction unless we stop purchasing these foods and demand change.

A lot of people are unaware, or care less, about the saga around sugar, and so find themselves in an oblivious state of over-consumption. That is until their friend, the "Pancreas" becomes insensitive, and the start of a gradual down-spiraling level of health will begin to change and wake up their lives.

I am not attacking sugar in general here, because we need sugar for survival, but we are exploring here the evils around artificial sugars because they are the real *baddies* in your life that we need to stay away from. I am awaiting the day that these manufacturers will be held accountable, and we start to reverse our health status and claim back our ideal weight.

I have personally had a sweet tooth for all of my life. Back in the day in my dad's store, we were selling lots of different things, and one of them was candy. I had to help out at times after school, and selling candy was a guaranteed daily sale. Kids came from school with a craving and had to have something before dinner, preferably without mom finding out.

I was no different. I ate a lot of candy in my life, and I feel lucky now to not have had any health problems after eating all those sugars in those years. The only evidence of damage left behind are the several fillings in my teeth (*these toxic mercury fillings are now replaced with a harmless resin*). I have learned my lesson, but still continue to satisfy my sugar cravings, only this time in a much healthier way. And that brings me to the heart of this step, and that is this:

!YOU NEED SUGAR—YOU ARE SUGAR!

It is the fuel for our cells and brain, and we need to daily supply ourselves. I can imagine that you are relieved now as maybe you were afraid that I would be recommending to forget about all sugar and leave it alone. Yes and no. We need sugar, but we need the *right type* of sugar in a correct balance with the fat intake in our diets (*please reread this last sentence*). I will show you how to responsibly satisfy your cravings without feeling bad and gaining weight (*even though some people do not crave sugar, see page 192*).

The average person in the modern world is eating roughly a scary 130 pounds or 59 kilos of the crystalline stuff in a year. That is about 50 teaspoons a day!! This is easily consumed when taking into account that it is everywhere, and knowing what the average person's diet consists of. We all know what the typical sugar sources are, but are you aware of the hidden sugars? The manufacturers in their greedy scam have also been hiding the sugar in apparently innocent foods.

Let's have a look at a few hidden sources of refined sugar:

- ⟩ Bread
- ⟩ Peanut butter
- ⟩ Pasta sauces
- ⟩ Fruit jams
- ⟩ Salad dressings
- ⟩ Granola bars
- ⟩ Fruit drinks
- ⟩ Canned veggies
- ⟩ Yogurt

In canned vegetables? Yep! But we have to stay away from all canned foods anyway as a small percentage still contains the dangerous BPA (*now replaced with other chemicals, BPS and BPF. Still harmful in my book*). Choose a glass jar. Look out for any syrups listed, mostly, "high fructose corn syrup." As you now know, bread is not a healthy food, even more so now because it also contains processed sugar. It's funny really, that people still fear the sugar in a single banana or mango because of weight-gain, but consuming processed foods fearlessly! More proof, of course, that the food propaganda machine is doing its job. I also have countless times observed people drinking a "diet soda" with a *high caloric* fatty meal. Fooled into believing that they are protecting themselves from weight-gain. I understand the power of adverts that the food industry uses on consumers, but this still gets me.

I want to give you a clearer understanding of how bad these fake sugars in processed foods are. Once this is established, we will focus on creating a renewed trust in natural sugars from whole foods, because natural sugar in itself is no direct health obstacle. "Do natural sugars make me gain weight?" An understandable and legitimate question, so let's continue exploring, as this is an important worry to tackle. But I wish to enlighten you first with an important insight:

"All the foods that you consume, and it does not matter what it is, will be converted by the body into sugar"

Refined or processed sugar is unnatural fragmented sugar. It is chemically and mechanically treated, and then heated so that nothing remains but pure addictive sweetness. It becomes a "refined crystallized carbohydrate." An amazing sixty-four food elements are destroyed in this process. So table sugar, in all its different shapes and forms, becomes a health hazard of the first rank. As for the syrups, like molasses, maple, honey, agave, brown rice, they are heated in their process as well, and the nutritional imbalances they create are ample.

Fortunately, we live in an era with great innovations where the health food industry is listening. Raw syrups are available now (*special machines do not heat the syrup*), and although they are still a concentrated sweetness, it is the better choice if you have to use sugar in your drink or elsewhere.

Glucose, or energy units, are the end product of digestion and assimilation. The healthiest path to obtain these needed elements is in the shortest possible route,—by eating fruit. Instead of taking a long and tiresome *backroad* by eating unnatural foods that require a laborious digestion by the body. In our energy creation, we rely on the ATP molecule or "Adenosine Triphosphate." It is the element that fuels the muscles by forming energy from the glucose molecule. And when muscles are exercised, sugar is better utilized (*page 58*).

When the body's rhythms and complex mechanisms are running correctly, an amazing intelligence will be at work. For example, the body knows exactly how many calories it needs and when/where they are required. When your eating instincts are restored, and you continue to eat natural foods, you will no longer overeat. The calories you'll eat from then on will be perfectly utilized to maintain all your essential bodily functions. To give you an idea:

- Body heat control
- Muscle movement
- Cell metabolizing
- Toxin removal
- Organ maintenance
- Weight-control

The body will then not store calories as fat anymore to all those unwanted places because there are no more excess calories to deposit. BUT, *blood-pumping exercise* needs to be included here as a vital lifestyle ingredient for this to work efficiently. "No pain—No gain," as they say.

Do you hear what I am saying here? Aim for a finely tuned machine—your body—and there will be no excess weight on you. The result of this *fine-tuning* will be a surplus of energy, which will lead to a desire to exercise and build a physically strong new you. The quest to find your *original* or *natural* health will become your goal in life. And as a bonus, your days of "Yo-Yo" dieting will be finally over.

The complicated part of this ideal weight controlling and perfect utilization of resources is controlled by a challenging mechanism that everybody has a different setting for. This bio-device can be called the "Fat-o-Stat." Like your home's thermostat, this regulator controls the fat stored by the body. Luckily, its setting to burn or store fat can be reset. A person's genetic predisposition plays a significant role in how this mechanism becomes set over the years. Its setting can totally frustrate a person when not able to lose or gain any weight despite all efforts. The brain controls this gauge, and it will calculatedly and endlessly defend its setting when you do not make a notable effort to change it.

This *fat-o-stat* does two things. Firstly, it will control the amount of food that you eat, influencing your appetite as needed. Second, it will control your energy expenditure to conserve or burn more as it sees fit. The key to *fooling* this intelligence is to increase exercise. When your caloric intake is higher than the amount burnt through activities, you cannot lower your setting. Many overweight people can eat only a 1000 calories a day and remain the same because they have trained their body to survive on little. This is the same with thin people who can eat tons of food and never gain weight.

Adjusting your fat-o-stat takes conscious effort that needs to be worked on for a prolonged time (*aging changes your setting too*). If you desire a different weight and physical shape, you will, with motivation and dedication, be able to reset your body's internal workings and mechanisms. The type and intensity of workout needed are personal, so you will need the guidance of a professional health educator/trainer who is familiar with this philosophy. Please visit my *website* to find out how I can help you to succeed.

I would like to take the opportunity here to emphasize the importance of *exercise*. Unfortunately, a lot of us still have a sedentary lifestyle that does not support a healthy human frame. Exercise is key to maintaining a healthy you because we are active animals by nature. We are designed to uphold muscle strength and tone. "When was the last time that you worked up a sweat?" Thirty minutes to a full hour a day will have your blood pumping actively through your system, and nothing will make you feel more alive!

Imagine every cell in your body being exercised while doing a cardiovascular workout. You will be able to bathe your cells in nutrients and clean house with fresh oxygen.

There is no better way to increase toxin removal and renewed cell metabolism than through exercise. We kinda know this, but we still need to be reminded that we have to keep on moving. It being stretching, aerobics, or weight training. On top of all that, it also helps you to "de-stress" by pumping that blood and increasing oxygen flow. Tone those muscles and regain your posture to help you feel good about yourself.

> *"What is more 'Attractive' than a toned body on a confident personality?"*

A new health path is not possible without a decent amount of movement in your life. Schedule your busy daily life to include a workout. Join a gym, walking club, yoga, swim, or start playing football, whatever it takes, just "do it!"

We are told how bad sugar is for our teeth,—but is it? We need to distinguish the important difference between natural and unnatural sugars. Your whole skeleton, including your teeth, are at risk when consuming these *unnatural* sugars. All refined sugars are extremely acid-forming. And as I explained with dairy products, all acidifying foods promote a leaking of the needed *acid buffering* calcium from your skeleton. Years of abuse can expose you to one of the most well-known bone weaknesses called osteoporosis, which is a scary prospect.

Because of these imbalances, the teeth can also become weak and more prone to developing cavities. It is not due to sugar being in contact with the teeth, but because your system has, again, become acidic, including your bones and teeth.

I tell you honestly that my teeth sensitivity has gone away ever since adopting the *raw food diet*, and I am eating plenty of fruit sugars. I presented this philosophy to a dentist once about to remove a very old tooth that was beyond saving (*a victim of my candy days*). He felt that it was not related. But then why would he agree? He needs people to eat harmful sugars for his livelihood, like doctors need sick people!

On a side note—I would like to stress that brushing your teeth is still a good idea after a fruit meal (*especially after any dried fruit, as it sticks to your teeth*). Brush your teeth only with some warm water (*toothpaste is toxic*) or eat a vegetable to naturally clean the teeth. At least, rinse your mouth with water, or with your own saliva. After a clean eating period, bad mouth odor will be a thing of the past, because you never know when a pair of lips are coming your way to kiss you.

Diabetes—We all know this one too well. This disease has started to reach an exponential number of victims. In the past, statistics would show that only people of middle age and older are at risk. But this has changed now! The age of contracting "Type II" diabetes is getting increasingly younger (*this is, of course, linked to obesity among children and young adults*). Babies and toddlers are now even at risk for contracting "Type I" or called "juvenile diabetes," as it is the most common chronic disease in children. Type I produces no insulin or very poorly, and daily insulin injections need to be followed for the rest of a person's life.

A pound of fruit like apples is about 270 calories, whereas one pound of candy is around 1800 calories. The body is not equipped to handle soo much sugar. You might think: "That's a lot of candy," but with today's *junk food* in our sugared society, a person could be eating this much or even more. The difference is also, as you now know, that the apple contains water and fiber, but the candy is pure refined sugar and so a direct onslaught on the sensitive pancreas insulin production.

Again, *artificial* sugars are detrimental for true health, and so diabetes has become in our western world one of the most frequent killers, after cancer and cardiovascular diseases.

Why and how diabetes is created is complex, and it would bore most readers, so let me give you the process in a nutshell (*this would also take several pages that would make this book too extensive*). Insulin helps to carry the sugar to its cells and regulates your blood sugar levels by lowering it when it is too high. This task is usually handled without any hiccups. The right balance between sweet sugar and fat is of the utmost importance here. You remember the analogy I gave you about your electric car making its way to its destination? When too much fat is consumed, and the blood becomes crowded with fat molecules, insulin production builds up, and your blood sugar levels drop onsetting an insensitivity. (*"hypoglycemia" is the first warning sign that something is up*). So, it is important to consume only natural sugars (*whole fruits*) and minimize fat intake. Refined fats and sugar are not allowed to dance together, so they need to be kept separated.

Please note that when eating only natural whole sugars and an excessive amount of natural fat, badly combined, can possibly still create the same issue,—but less likely. Natural fat and sugar are easier assimilated by the system and do not obstruct. What follows is a list of possible health challenges that a person can encounter if not careful with sugar and fat.

- ➢ Toxic acid body
- ➢ Organ dysfunctions
- ➢ Hypoglycemia
- ➢ Diabetes
- ➢ Emotional instability
- ➢ Mental illness
- ➢ Heart disease
- ➢ Weight gain

We have come now to the "soul" of this steps philosophy:

"The healthiest way to fully energize our amazing bodies is with natural simple sugars,—Carbohydrates"

And we need to obtain these from whole food sources, the way only nature can provide them. When these right foods are consumed, we will manifest real unspoiled health because the body can operate uninhibited. Remember that we need to maintain enough energy to handle bodily tasks with an energy-*saving* digestion and avoid energy-*draining* practices, like eating difficult to digest foods, stress, poor sleep, or overexertion. The glucose from our Earthly delights will go straight to the cells for energy as no detour for digestion is needed, there are no obstacles. Athletes have now discovered the power that a banana, for example, can deliver to them. There is just no yummier "natural energy" source.

All this talk about sugar and real nourishment reminds me of a story that happened to me many years ago. A lady I had been consulting about health and nutrition mentioned that she wanted to bring along her daughter next time. She was in college abroad and would be coming home for Christmas. "My daughter [she started telling me] is at the troublesome young age of nineteen and has been for the whole of her life, pretty much, eating jam sandwiches. That is the only thing she likes to eat." She fought many battles to have her daughter eat vegetables and fruit. Hearing this, I was shocked and said that I would be very curious to talk to her. At the same time, I thought how poor her health must be and how dreadful she must look for not having any real nutrition for all those years. All these processed sugars combined with white bread will seriously stress the pancreas and create all sorts of issues.

I could have known about the surprise that awaited me when I finally met the girl. In walked this tall teenager with beautiful red hair, a big smile, and flawless white skin. I was immediately reminded of the resilience of young bodies and the onslaught we can take at that age. No poor nutrition was evident, but I still expressed my concern. She said that she had taken joy, since in college, in eating various other things. But, oh my, that revelation did not change anything because she still did not eat any fruits or greens.

Appearances can be really deceiving. Even though no consequences were visible on this young maiden due to her youth's advantage, her health is still suffering silently. If she does not change, she most likely will start to feel the effect of poor nutrition in years to come. Her advantage has its limits. So, although you can survive on bread and jam, you are inevitably breaking many important nutritional laws.

When in Transition

Allow me to mention again,—"we need sugar, we are sugar!" So, let's look at sugar from a positive angle and get rid of our sugar fears, as we need to fuel our amazing machine.

The first important step that needs to be taken is to eliminate the laboratory sweeteners from your life, as these, again, will create unhealthy cravings. Do away with all the artificial sugars in your kitchen, and all these little sachets of lab sugar that you carry with you to use when needed.

Then, a trip to the health food store to look for any raw sugars, in syrup or crystallized form, that will replace the chemical ones. If they do not carry any raw sugar brand, then the second option will be to get *regular* sugar. At this point, anything is better than the low-calorie artificial sweeteners.

A special note to "honey" as this nectar of the Gods (*it is bee vomit, to be honest here*) is not good either, sorry. I know many people swear by honey, but it also gets heated in its production process. So it becomes a dangerous sugar source that will mess with your pancreas. Okay, you also have raw honey, if you can find it, which will make the honey more natural to use. It is still a too concentrated sugar fix, but fine as a transition sugar. Careful though, as a conscious Vegan now (*they do not eat honey*), you could still eat too much of it. I think you get the picture. Make it a habit now to check for the sugar contents of any food you buy from now on and continue to lower your artificial sugar intake.

Also, try to replace your snack foods, like candy bars with dried bananas, apples, grapes, mango, or maybe some sweet "Medjool" dates,—yummy! When replacing *faux* sugars with real ones, you are on track for a new you.

My Cleaner Advice

Eat as much sugar as you desire. Sounds too good to be true, right? To a certain point, this is precisely what you can do. How would you feel about eating dessert pretty much all of the time? Okay, I know, I cannot turn you into a fruit eater just like that, but I do hope you will start to incorporate it a lot more in your daily diet. You will be amazed as to how great and clean it will make you feel.

Start to introduce more fruits into your life in the morning. Whatever your breakfast used to be, replace it slowly with more fruits. I know you will feel at first that it will not sustain you enough for your busy mornings, but I suggest to increase your portions every day. A large fruit smoothie is a great way for the active person to take in delicious fruit quickly.

Not that I really recommend rushing in the morning, but I am being realistic here. Think about the large variety of fruits that you can find in the markets today. You will never get bored. This clean path should be easy for you, as it is soo delicious.

Experiment with different fruits to find out which ones you like best and will sustain you. Personally, bananas are my best friends (*the king of fruits*) to get me through the biggest part of the day. Cut them up in a bowl, or blend them up to enjoy!

When you are ready to eat even cleaner than ever before, eating plenty of fruit should be your goal and the only sugar source in your life (*of course veggies and greens are onboard as well to alkalize and nourish*). And for protein, to be clear again, you have the nuts and seeds alongside the denser fruits.

To recap—Vegetables and greens can always be mixed with fruits. Nuts and seeds can always be mixed with veggies and greens, but nuts NOT with fruits. To avoid any digestive conflicts, try some of my "hygienic clean recipes" to keep things interesting (*see my website videos*).

When desiring a change, make a raw burger or any other raw gourmet dish for your evening meal. I am only being realistic because although you could feel totally satisfied with fruit every day, I understand that you want variety, and that's okay. Take your time with this. Let your instincts and desires guide you to what to eat. But be aware that this takes practice because undoubtedly, you will still have addictive *cooked food* habits lingering in your system. Specific cravings that will give you a false signal of what foods you wanna eat.

The two powerful instinctive signals to deal with every day are "true hunger and cravings." And it takes inner-balance and practice to recognize the seductive signals of the latter one.

Basically, when you are hungry, you will eat anything to silence that roaring lion (*start peeling those mangoes*). And when going through the craving signals, you will be looking for something more specific to eat. Usually, this will be a snack, cookie, or sweet candy of some kind.

If you eat enough nutrient-dense foods during a preferably proper sit-down meal, and the table is left feeling full and satisfied, cravings should not appear in-between meals. It is not easy in the beginning to determine what is what, so do your best to recognize which one is—talking to you.

I would like to share here a story that I followed in 2009 that I found particularly tragic. It was the ordeal of Patrick Swayze. You know, he got fame through the "Dirty Dancing" and "Ghost" movie. He got stage IV "pancreatic cancer" and was diagnosed with months to live. I was interested to learn about the medical world's treatment path and whether he would become better. But after a battle of twenty months, he died. He told the world that he would, "Kick it!" He kept on working and people applauded him for that. But unfortunately this heroic action was the wrong path to follow. He went on to use up all his *healing* energies by working and creating stress.

On top of it all, he kept on smoking, sad to say. I do not know what diet he followed, but I know that his loss could have been avoided most likely. He would have had a fairer chance of survival when he would have rested, fasted, ate real foods, and of course, stopped smoking and alcohol (*assuming that he drank*). By doing so, he would have respected the natural laws that we learned about in this book so far. Also, with him, the chemo did not work. He was told that his cancer was too far advanced to treat. A shame . . . a darn shame!

* * * * * *

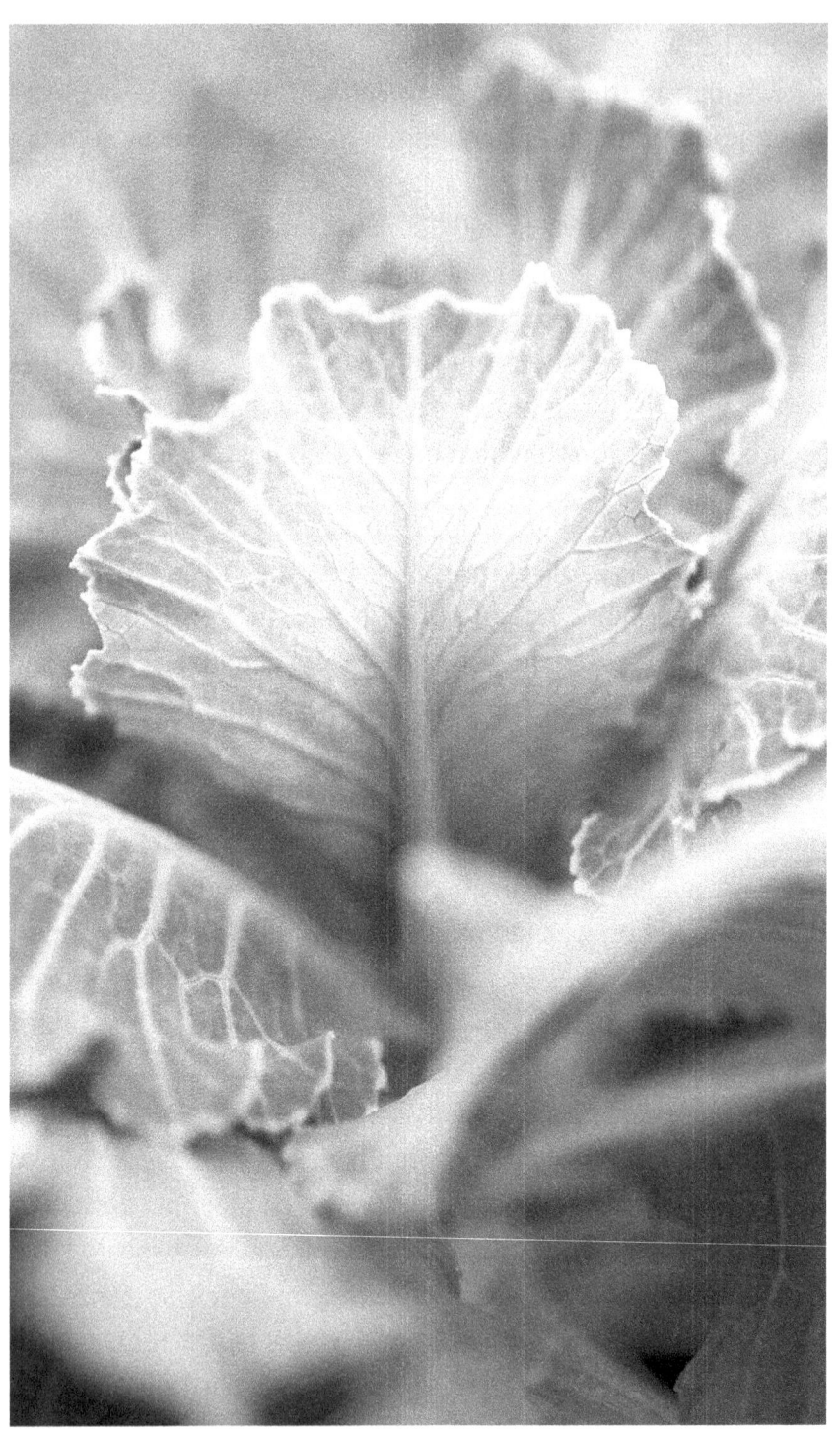

STEP
NUMBER EIGHT

ALCOHOL

Alcohol plays a much-needed part in our modern-day world, and it is at the same time a troublesome substance that creates much suffering. But despite its bad reputation, the cultural ritual of becoming inebriated still is, to a certain degree, acceptable behavior in our communities. You noticed that I wrote, "much-needed" in the first sentence, so let me explain.

Alcohol is everywhere. It has become a recreational drug that appears innocent and normal in most people's lives. In many cultures in the world, you better not dare to take it away, you would most likely start a civil war. Alcohol is "fun time" for some and destroying lives for others. In 1920 it became prohibited to drink alcohol in the United States, and it created much upheaval among the people. This ban was lifted 13 years later because the uproar and conflicts never stopped.

When I observe the world, I see the urgent need to be able to escape. As I mentioned in the *coffee step,* people have always felt the need to switch-off reality. Many people feel trapped in their lives and jobs, and their emotional state is often grim. These days real joy is a rare gem. When you talk to people, it becomes clear that most, if not all, are looking in their own way for a path to happiness. They wish to feel content in what they are doing and how they are being.

There is a lot of financial pressure in our societies! Which gets fueled even more by a stressful system mostly present in our large unnatural cities where people's true freedom is kept in check. Living this way creates a lot of unhealthy tension. Stress is always poisonous and, therefore, unhealthy to our sensitive constitution, and it is not supposed to be this way.

"I claim that presently our societies are set up wrong"

Physical and mental stress at work, on the street, in traffic, at home, on TV. There is no real escape from it, except maybe in a bottle of—booze. This is my personal view of the reason why people want to escape in alcohol (*or other drugs*). That said, I also believe that it is, to a certain degree, a savior to our very stressful world. If people had absolutely no way to run from the frustrations surrounding us, it all could be a lot worse. Alcohol is also ancient as it was even found inside the tombs of Pharaohs. So, the urge to dull and excite the mind and body has been around for quite some time now.

The fermentation process to produce commercial alcohol is a biochemical process similar to how the body's "microflora" converts carbohydrates into tiny amounts of *ethanol*. This occurs daily in your gut, and the body avoids a toxic buildup through a mechanism called, "catabolic degradation."

And when it comes to alcohol being created in our guts because of fruit fermentation, gastrointestinal experts say that this is a old myth. Because fermentation in the stomach is impossible because the strong stomach acids make life for a bacteria there pretty impossible, and with that, I agree. Food-combining is also a myth to these experts. They say that there are no issues at all with just randomly consuming food.

Well, I personally, and other fellow fruit eaters I talked to feel the conflict when not being careful with foods, sorry experts! I still say that you can create a funky smelling acidic stomach *soup* that will result in an unclean, toxic system when not careful. With its non-foods, our modern world is plagued with all kinds of chronic gastrointestinal disorders, like various degrees of "acid reflux." So, how are these then created? Causes for reflux do vary, but the advice given by doctors to remedy this is usually to be careful with food. I need to express that some professionals do not see the big picture. They often diagnose without considering a patient's diet, let alone a much cleaner way of eating, as I recommend. So, it seems clear to me that just *downloading* anything you like is bad practice. Pay attention and learn from your body!

Commercial alcohols will play with your health. It is like salt, a protoplasmic poison that kills at the cellular level. All organs are affected by alcohol. After continuous abuse, the central nervous and cardiovascular system, gastrointestinal tract, liver, and kidneys will become weakened and start to gradually decline in function. But, I am not only talking about the consequences of a lifetime of abuse, like that of an alcoholic (*clearly, a daily drinker will have a shorter route to this self-destruction*). No one is never really exempt from alcohol effects, even when only having two drinks a week.

A worrying result in the world of frequent drinkers is the chemical imbalances that one creates when intoxicating the body. The blueprint of our Earthly creation is easily thrown off balance when boundaries are pushed beyond their limits. An imbalanced chemical brain can do all kinds of things to you. Depression is, in many cases, the unpleasant outcome of frequent drinking and often results in the ruining of families. Also, violent tendencies can be released in a person tearing loved ones apart. It is all good fun to have a drink with your friends in a bar, but it should be a laugh in moderation. But then moderation has a different meaning for everybody.

Alcohol in your system on a night of binging can *kill* about 100,000 brain cells. It constricts your arteries, raises your blood pressure, and weakens the liver. Let's see what effects can be created when abusing this recreational drug:

- Dehydration
- Constriction of the arteries
- Kills cells on contact
- Raises blood pressure
- Loss of potassium
- Damage to heart muscles
- Mental illnesses
- Cirrhosis of the liver
- Digestive problems
- Poor nutrient absorption

Our bodies are self-repairing, maintaining, and healing, but only within their limits, though. When given the opportunity, specific damage can be repaired, but maybe not always to its original state. Cirrhosis of the liver is a good example. When the liver's sensitive tissues become damaged by the alcohol, the body will start to repair them as well as it can. Usually, however, the tissues will be replaced with *scarred* ones and the crucial tasks of the liver will become challenged.

And let's not forget, as listed above, that excessive alcohol intake can cause "hypertension." High blood pressure kills many people yearly. It puts a strain on various organs and blood vessels, hence, weakening the heart muscle.

It is a killer! I know that sounds very dramatic, but what else wakes a person up to what could be destroying their precious gift of health? People do not seem to be fully aware of the consequences like you also see with smoking. It is puzzling to me now (*I quit in 1993*) when I see a person still grabbing two packs of the shelf in the supermarket after all those many years of information to the public. Even now, with massive words on a pack of cigarettes saying: "Smoking will KILL you!" Okay, you are a teenager, and you need to look cool, but smoking as an adult? It's a very addictive habit (*contains ± 4000 chemicals to keep you smoking*), and I really understand that it is not easy to quit. Even so, it still perplexes me that smoking still continues after a so-called wiser age.

I do not want to sound condescending here, but plenty of adults can really behave like kids. They also need to grow up into a world with consequences. If it is alcohol, cigarettes, cigars, or any other bad habit, they do not seem to care. I know that these issues go a lot deeper than that, but still, on the surface it appears illogical and immature. As you can tell, this is frustrating to me because we need to move on as a dignified human race. We have to leave sickness behind and clean up our act.

"It is time for suffering to end!"

Us growing up as a species is a process. But where is the logic in continuing to destroy our precious health when we know better, as these vices take many lives every year? But our greedy governments are largely responsible as well as they permit the selling of alcohol and cigarettes. Is it because they make tons of money from their sales, or do they really fear that they will have real riots on their hands when banned?

I envision a far Utopian future where it is being displayed in a history museum, of whatever technology they will have, the era we live in now. And what is shown is our global use of a little stick loaded with chemicals being used to burn tobacco that we inhale. Together with chronic alcohol consumption and harmful chemical drugs that have the destructing task in poisoning all our healthy cells. I already see those people in the future shake their heads in disbelieve as in how stupid and primitive we were then.

Alcoholic fluids will destroy that which gives life. There is a dark cloud hanging over many households, as many kids are already the victims of a drunken society. It all seems a bit innocent at first glance and I wish that the frequent drinkers of alcohol would recognize its downfalls because when you look deep into the bottle, many disillusions you will find.

When in Transition

I have no suggestions here, only some more sensible (*I hope*) advice. I know how much fun an evening in a bar can be, and I can only suggest minimizing your intake. Try to say: "NO!" when a new round of drinks is being ordered. An occasional glass of wine or a bottle of beer is okay when it is consumed in good fun. We all want to forget our busy stressful week for one evening and "paint the town red" with our girlfriends or buddies, but it does not need to be abusive.

What also helps is to change the alcohol that you drink and to go easy on the hard liquor. No judgments here, but throwing back shots and playing drinking games are the fun practices of a teenager. After a certain age, it does not look cool anymore (*not saying that it is ever cool*). Wine and beer fall in the maybe more *innocent* category, although it is possible to drink lots of those as well. As a reminder, alcohol poisoning is a real thing, and people, young and old, have died from it. Sometimes it just gets more serious than only needing a bucket next to your bed.

When I became raw in 2013, I still had my "party Devil" on my shoulder telling me to have a drink or three. I resorted to only drinking fermented grapes as it is technically raw. Wine is not cooked like the grains in beer and liquor. Wine is also free of the problematic gluten we talked about in this book.

Luckily, I was never a big drinker because I always hated it to feel sick. In time you will find that the cleaner you become, the lesser the desire for alcohol.

Also here, take your time to slowly minimize your intake. And when you have your party pals from the good old days banging on the door for a night of boozing, maybe it is time for them to take a new direction or leave you out of the fun.

There are other options to look into that you might find enjoyable. Sports are a great way to unwind. Mediation and listening to music are also inspiring outlets to clear stress from your being. Another way to prevent drinking alcohol is to talk about it in confidence to somebody. People can quickly accumulate frustrations that can result in depression or anger to then only find alcohol as their savior. This behavior has been tried. It does not work to hold stuff in. So, go ahead and do some *soul searching* and find another escape route.

My Cleaner Advice

Let's be honest, to not drink in a bar with your friends or at a business party is still a "feeling-out-of-place" situation. These are some of the social obstacles you will have to overcome because when desiring an energetic clean body, a complete abstinence of alcohol needs to be followed. Stand your ground when facing disbelief and maybe even ridicule at the hands of people. It is cliché behavior and very boring!

Give yourself the needed time to completely detox, as the cleaner you become, the more you will resent the poisonous effect of alcohol. It is not the end of the world if you have a small glass of wine or beer once on a full moon if it will not lead to drinking more. Act according to your self-control.

* * * * * *

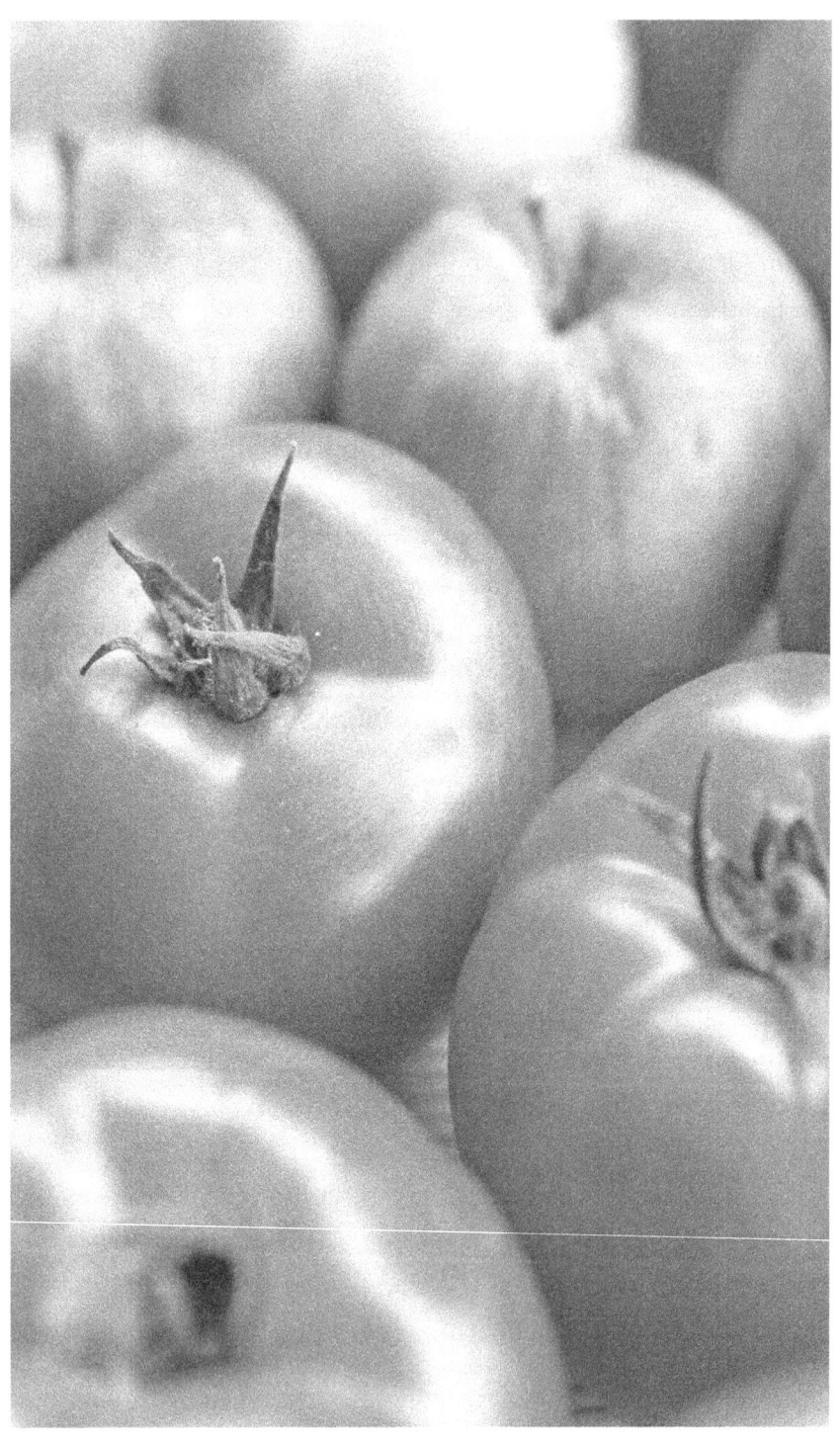

STEP
NUMBER NINE

WATER

I have been waiting eagerly to write this *step* because I find the topic of water extremely fascinating. To start, I am not pointing a bad finger at water in general here because we all know that we cannot live without water. Water is mysterious, to say the least, and I will make an attempt to reveal some of its secrets to you. Hopefully, you will understand why we not only need to watch what water we drink but also what we think and say, as we are made mostly of water.

All the previous *steps* involved removing the identified ingredient in our lives, and I am also doing this with water. I will be pointing out several varieties of "unstructured" water we have in our lives. This water has no real health benefits. It has become like processed foods, a denatured substance that has lost its lifeforce. It is essential that we surround ourselves with quality water, to make sure that we drink, eat (*fruits and vegetables*), or wash ourselves with this life-giving molecule, which happens to be our—"birthright."

It is also of utmost importance that we maintain a sacred connection with our water. Connection? Well, let me first say that some of the insights I will be sharing with you might come over as strange or too-far-out-there as they say. But life is undoubtedly much more mysterious than we think it is. So, I suggest to keep an open mind and allow this fascinating information to enter your life because we find out new truths every day that were ridiculed the day before.

"Water, the great mystery" is a documentary that I highly recommend. It is about our symbiosis with water and its perplexing properties. This liquid of life is the most essential ingredient when one seeks radiant health. That our planet and bodies consist roughly of 70% percent water and the fact that we cannot live without this element should be a clue. Water has been here since it all started. Life sprung from water, of this you are aware, but what most people do not know is that water has a memory, yes indeed, a,—memory!

It has its *original structure* in its memory, as in how it was organized at the very beginning. Water, in its original design, like your health, is the most potent of all waters. It is water with all its life-creating and mystical properties intact. Pure clean water is susceptible to many negative influences, and its environment for one affects it profoundly.

Water rains down on us from the heavens in a "hexagonal" structured state, meaning it is not polluted or contaminated in any way (*this is how it is initially designed*). You have learned that when a natural element is in order, it will be able to interact with other elements. Do you think that life could have been created in the perfection that it is in if the elements of life were just a bundle of distorted unorganized molecules? The Universe, in all its chaotic appearance, is a natural order. Thus, there is a natural order within you.

Water holds the memory of who we are. Crazy, I know, but this has been established (*water memory documentary*). The person behind this fascinating data is Luc Montagnier, a virologist, and researcher. He and his team discovered the human HIV virus, so he comes with impressive credentials. As far-fetched these new theories are for some people, they shape a vital view on life itself that will help us in the future.

Water in its uncorrupted original state, so with its memory intact, will continue to bring beautiful life to our planet and its inhabitants forever. Unless we mess it up completely.

So, water in its purest form has not only all the ingredients to create life but it has also the intelligence within its structure to maintain its own blueprint. To preserve "natural order" since the birth of the Universe. We are many billions of years separated from the creation of our planet's water and most certainly, since we humans arrived and started our industrial revolution, our water has gone through many transformations.

In physics, it is still a puzzling question of why water is the only substance on the planet that can exist in three states of matter: "Liquid, Solid, and Gaseous." And this is not where the intriguing questions stop. A renowned Russian scientist's brave statement is that the scientific world still does not know anything about water.

With the start of our industrial revolution, somewhere in the 1800s, a major contributor to our present waters alteration was born. Our ancient water has since changed,—and not for the better! It is safe to say that water is losing its *original programming* only because of us humans. This decline of its structural integrity has everything to do with pollution. Our waters are transforming because we are dumping all our dangerous chemicals in it (*industrial and household*).

It is expressed repeatedly that our arrogance has led us to the polluting of our Mother Earth. The notion that we can do anything we want for the benefit of progress. The insane damage caused to our life-giving world for the purpose of making money is a haunting dark nightmare. As I mentioned before, our evolution as a species needs time, it is a process, but will we ever learn is the question.

The list of what is being done to our beautiful blue planet, the only home we have, by the way, is long:

- ☠ Factories
- ☠ Chemical laboratories
- ☠ Agriculture
- ☠ Livestock breeding
- ☠ Genetic manipulation
- ☠ Nuclear fusion
- ☠ Combustion engines
- ☠ Industrial and household chemicals
- ☠ Oil drilling and spilling
- ☠ Fracking
- ☠ Chemtrails

All these continue to "destroy" our precious Ecosystem, and at the center is the polluting of our beautiful waters.

Everything is linked together, and we can only prosper as a species when the elements around us are healthy and in order. All the man-made chemical components not recognized by nature will end up, like inside your body, creating toxins and serious imbalances in nature's intricate fabric. Ironically, technological advancements made it possible to design the tools to examine these damages, properly assess them, and create changes. It is happening this cleaning up of our act, but way to slow if you ask me. The political corruption and bureaucratic red tape are as always slowing real progress down. Personally, I do not see the point of conducting endless research to find out that we are destroying our planet. It is clear as water that something is not right with our home, and we all need to act—yesterday!

Water and life is a miracle. It starts for us already at an early stage that water becomes so important as it is in the "amniotic fluid" in the womb where our growth occurs. Did you know that the amniotic bag is mostly water? I say mostly because after about 16 weeks, or so, when the fetal kidneys start to function, the baby's urine will also be part of this important amniotic sac. This life-giving water holds all the nutrients, hormones, and antibodies the fragile baby needs. This watery fluid also protects the baby from possible outside bumps and keeps the temperature constant for a comfortable growing environment. The fluid also helps the development of the digestive system, lungs, muscles, and bones. So, you see that water is where we come from. Water is that essential element in our first nine months and on our path to becoming human. Throughout our lives, we feel protected, nourished, and comforted by water. Various water therapy practices exist nowadays, helping people restore their physical and mental health through this mysterious liquid's healing abilities.

I want to mention the work of the late Dr. Emoto Masaru. He is said to have discovered that when water is exposed to specific emotions, it changes its physical form. He had many people for the first time in awe about what he found in the documentary: "What the Bleep Do We Know!?" When, e.g., water was exposed to kind and harsh words, or classical and hard rock music, a water's structure would change. When examined under a special microscope, a beautiful crystallized design would be observed when kindness and gentleness were expressed (*much like snowflakes*), and a dark and ugly one when violence and aggression were used.

In the water documentary, they conducted very fascinating laboratory tests with bottles of unstructured or "ugly" water that gets blessed by a priest. This water became completely structured (*religion plays no role here, it's all about the kind intentions*). Thoughts and words are energy, and energy influences mass (*this is a scientific fact*). This experiment showed that those drops of perfect water held the memory of beauty and perfection and passed it on to the unstructured ugly water. Some people call this pseudoscience, you decide.

All the foods that we grow for consumption contain high amounts of water, even a seemingly dry carrot holds a lot of liquid. The essentials for growing are not only the soil and the sunshine, but also the water that rains down from the sky. Our water is then evaporated into the air where the droplets gather together and form clouds until it gets too crowded. After, they all fall back to the Earth as rain to bring renewed lifeforce to everything. All water in nature is "vortex-ed." It moves in a spiral motion. You can see this in natural bodies of water, like rivers and streams, wherever water in nature is in movement. With this moving action, it is charging and structuring itself with the energies emanating from our planet. It becomes understandable then that only this life-giving water should be given to seeds to grow our foods.

Talking about vitalizing water. I have observed the practice of seeds to be planted being put in a person's mouth first so that they mix with the saliva to come to know the farmer's intentions. In Costa Rica, where I worked at a health farm that grows their own organic fruits and greens, I witnessed an unusual way to let the seeds get acquainted with the land—and its new owners. They bought pasture land and were told by the locals that you cannot grow anything on that type of soil. Well, all their fruit trees are thriving in every possible way. The reason for sharing this, they collect their personal waste from an alive raw food diet and mix it with the soil that feeds all their young fruit trees and plants. Besides the added nutrition, their urine and feces hold the information and their sincere intentions for the land. Too far out for you maybe, but it worked for them.

I did a well-known experiment once where I had two almonds that I wanted to sprout. I put each of them in a little jar with soil and poured over one some fresh rainwater, and over the other rainwater I had microwaved for 30 seconds. The first almond started to show a little tail after a few days, but the other one just started to rot in the soil I planted it in. We can agree that life is mysterious, but to see this enigma in action is a whole other thing.

Food and water are intertwined in the structure of life. The human species are therefore interconnected with our natural food sources and all other lifeforms. "Life-giving" foods contain the original structured water that works like a battery charged by the sun's infrared rays for energetic health.

Those of us living in the modern western world have our water pumped up to our houses. It has its origin at the water treatment plant where it is filtered and chemically treated. Next, the water gets pumped through a vastly complex system of pipes and delivered to your faucet, such convenience. The problem here is not only that the water has to be treated, but also that it is transported through a pipe system that does not allow it to be recharged. We are unfortunately interacting with water which original design is being destroyed.

Then we have "Chlorine Dioxide, Chlorite, and 'Hydrofluorosilicic Acid" (*a hazardous chemical from the fertilizer industry*), used in our water treatment plants! Adding these chemicals for safer drinking water is just absurd (*but a necessary evil in today's polluted world*). It is killing the environment and—you! Then WE use it for food preparation, cleaning house/car, and bathing, where even more destruction takes place in the form of heating/microwaving, household chemicals, and the use of chemical body products.

Here we have water that is supposed to give us life and health, doing the opposite. Try to cook your food less and eat fresh whenever you can. Also, I strongly suggest doing away with your microwave oven if you have one, as it is simply a dangerous machine. I always say that if manufacturers called those ovens for what they truly are, which is a "radiation" oven, nobody would buy them.

When we cook our foods, we are not only doing harm by removing its water and vitamin/nutrient contents, but also by changing its molecular structure. Our kitchens, with all their modern-day appliances, are indeed like chemical laboratories. Irreversible damage is done when manipulating our natural foods, whether on the stove, in the oven, or by radiation.

"Water is life,—heat or fire is death"

It is all pretty simple really.

Another fantastic part of the properties of water, besides the memory, is its role in healing. As a "Hygienic Doctor" I love learning about the intricacies of life. The mysterious intelligence of nature, and therefore of our bodies. We learn, contrary to popular belief that no substance or influence of any kind can directly instigate healing, that,

"Only the body has the lifeforce to do so"

People still believe that a doctor's pill or a hot cup of herbal tea will cure us of our ailments. There is truly nothing that comes out of the pharmacy, nor what granny once used, that can directly overwrite the body's infinite intelligence. Even an organic apple cannot do that. It is actually an insult to the intelligence of the Universe to think that creation is imperfect and that we need to assist it with a man-made concoction or natural substance. We need to regain our trust in nature.

When observing our water, it becomes evident that it is responsible, directly or indirectly, for our well-being. If it is the purity of our drinking water, the water in our organic produce, water in a recreational and relaxing capacity, or the actual positive views one has. When learning about these many extraordinary water capabilities, it is then a "no-brainer" to see that we need to respect the water within us and in our environment. When we realize that our bodily water elements can influence our health, we ought to be more careful. Not only about what we consume, but also give attention to our thoughts (*still a controversial idea*).

You can eat fruits and greens all you want, but if you are most of the time stressed and angry with a negative attitude towards life, then all those delights are not going to give you amazing health. I have rarely though come across a negative fruit/veggie eater, but to be fair here, there are many poor diet consumers that are pretty positive too. Impossible, of course, to put a solid finger on the facts in these assumptions. So based on these amazing observations about water, I feel certain that we are positively influenced by the water in our organic produce (*pesticides and herbicides can form toxic chemical bonds in the brain*). We need to conclude that our beautiful pristine nature is a perfect "living system," as everything indicates this to be so. Therefore, it is beyond essential that the world "comes to its senses again" and starts working WITH what gives us life, instead of working against it. We have to STOP polluting our waters! Please help this cause in any way you can. Thanks.

"It's time for a '(R)evolution,' so the natural world can heal!"

In the NH philosophy, we learn that nature has its laws in place, and they need to be respected if you choose the path of "Original Health." We need to trust her infinite wisdom and treasure her in all her beauty and wonder, because,—where would we be without Mama Nature?

When in Transition

The transition I am suggesting here is to watch your water intake. Take some time to investigate the water that you have in your immediate environment. Go to your water provider for more details, or send a sample to a lab where they will assess the quality of the water you have coming into your home. It is important to know.

I suggest giving up on buying bottled water if you are doing so. Bottled water is extremely bad for the environment as all these plastic bottles are just piling up on our garbage dumps and in our oceans. Recycling is happening, but still. Bottled water can be a scam, as water companies have been caught bottling tap water. Also, store-bought water contains leaked toxins from the plastics. But the store and the water company are not the only sources to get water from. If you are lucky enough, you can find a groundwater well (*have the water tested!*). Maybe there is even one in your back garden, so it is time to take out your "Dowsing rod."

You have all kinds of filters on the market these days (*kitchen and shower*). Depending on where you are located, they can be a necessary investment. Another recommended gadget to own is a "structure-izer." Which you can buy to put between your water pipes, which will *recharge* the water by vortexing it inside the device itself. Also, a water distiller powered by the almighty sun could be a must have for you (*regular machines boil the water, but you do not need to boil to distill*). It will remove all the impurities. After making several liters/gallons, you can pour it in large glass bottles to be placed outside to let the sun and moon revitalize it again. You can even add some lemon juice to help with the process. It's all a bit of work, but so worth it in the end. It is in your hands to implement these suggestions. I just hope that from now on, you will see your water in a whole new puddle.

My Cleaner Advice

For us cleaner people on the planet, it is all a lot simpler. If you eat a lot of fruit, you will have no real reason to drink water anymore. You rarely will become thirsty because of your high intake of structured water, and assuming no more salt and spices are consumed. So, bring your juicy fruits, and extra water with you when hiking or other sun activity, so you don't have to worry about dangerous dehydration.

One more thing, please forget about all those glasses of water that we are told to drink every day. Quench your need for liquids only when thirsty, because your body has no use for it when you are hydrated. Make sure that you pee, on average, at least eight times a day (*depending on climate, in hot weather you will perspire the water more*). "Clear pee" is the only true indicator that shows if you are hydrated or not and are cleaning your system. And when following a clean fruit diet, those many trips to the bathroom are—guaranteed.

* * * * * *

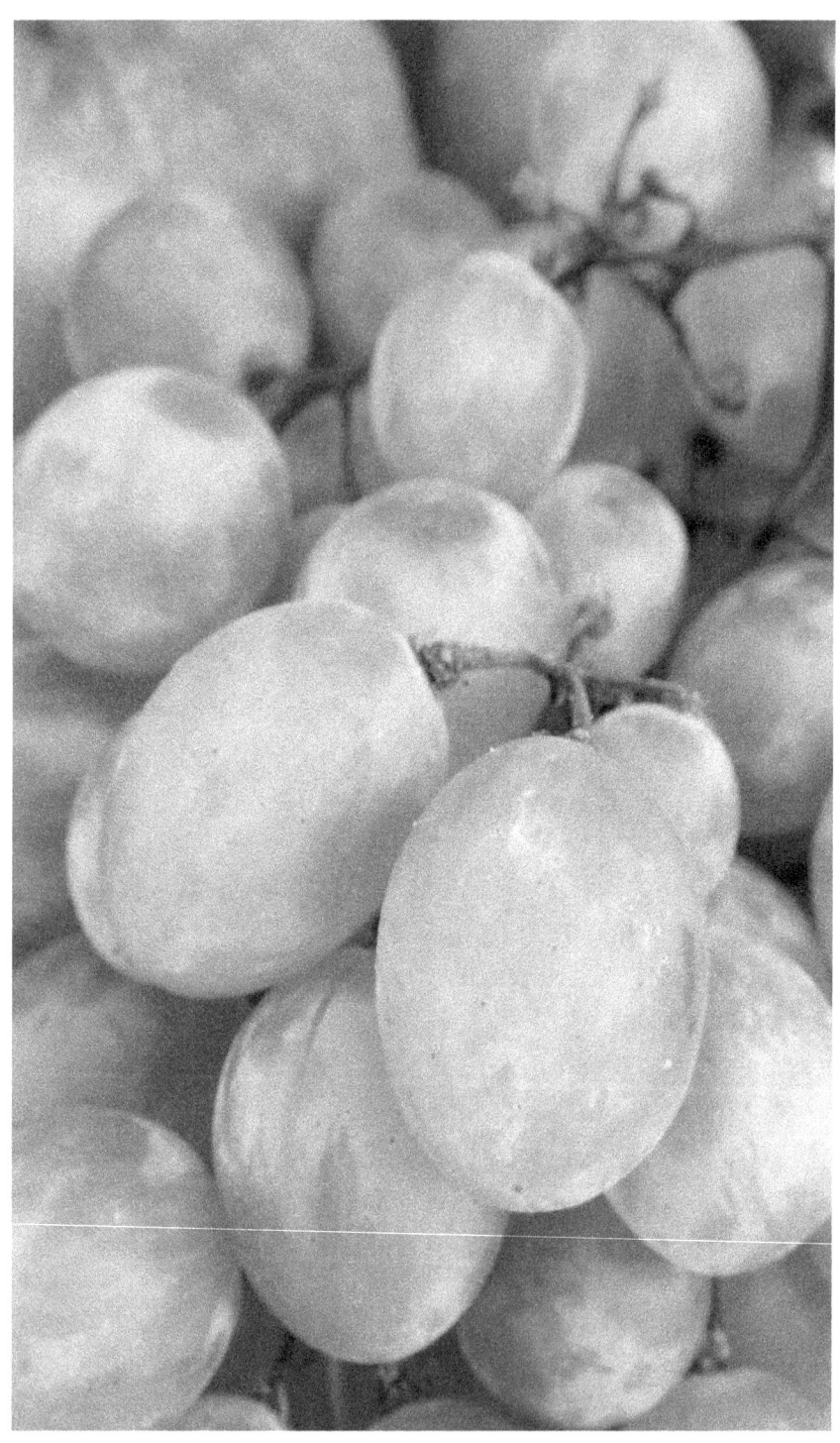

STEP
NUMBER TEN

ENVIRONMENT

And we have arrived at our very last *step*. Here I am not referring to our beautiful natural environment, of course, but the "artificial" one that many of us live in. We are going to take a look at your home environment. Because most likely, you have constant daily exposure to hidden toxins that can undoubtedly poison your health.

As we have learned, your body-environment is intricately linked to your outer-environment. It is designed this way because your natural environment needs to nourish your bio-machine for survival. An amazing symbiotic design really if you think about it. Your largest natural tool that connects you with your outer-surroundings is, obviously,—your skin. It has quite the surface area and many functions to complete on a daily basis. Not only does it keep you safe and protected, but also looking young as long as it can. This is something that most of us are after, right? We have accepted the fact that we grow in chronological age, but the physical aging, well, that is still a huge problem for many. It is observed that this aging issue is a bigger problem for our lovely ladies, hence the multi-billion valued beauty industry. But more men are now attempting to tackle "father time" the best they can as well.

There is a lot we can do, but it is a vast scam when we are told that you can find your *youth* again in a bottle of cream. As I have pointed out to you before, we always need to get to the root cause of a problem. Like in nature, it is a violation when a body's natural equilibrium is disrupted and changed through the use of unnatural toxic products. An innate force will then make an attempt to restore its original balanced state. Here, the law of *cause and effect* will attempt to restore "law and order," a construct to respect in our lives. Not only for your health and well-being but also for any other action in the physical world. So, let's cover a few health assaults that you can find in your immediate home environment so that you can sleep worry-free.

We have already covered the inside of our bodies, but now we need to have a magnified look at the direct outside of them, namely,—personal hygiene. We must maintain a high, but not obsessive, standard of cleanliness. A closer look at our daily ritual of cleansing is needed and the many outside forces that could disrupt this beautifying routine.

To recap—The philosophy of Natural Hygiene refers to our inner/outer cleanliness.

There is much to be said about beauty. It influences our everyday lives and our happiness on many levels. Beauty is everywhere, even in the perceived ugliness that surrounds us. Beauty is found in every little detail. Perfection is beauty. You will agree that we live in a society where appearance is important. That particular physical qualities can help you progress faster. Judgment is everywhere, and many souls suffer from this on a daily basis. People are ceaselessly being indoctrinated with a certain image on TV, in magazines, the Internet, and in public.

"Vitality and beauty are gifts of nature for those who live according to its laws"

- Leonardo da Vinci

If we believe the commercials (*we often do*), this beauty and eternal youth can be found in the form of a lotion or any other concoction. There is a real superficial aspect that plays in our society of beauty that produces a whole lot of unhappy and insecure people because they happen not to look like the persons in the magazine. This is a social issue that we are not going to talk about here, but it is still good to realize that these judgmental notions are going on.

"True beauty is only skin deep"

A well-known saying goes. Clearly, a person's values and character are more important than how he/she appears on the outside. And that's why I believe that if more people would follow our natural laws of life, so a more balanced connection with nature and a humane lifestyle, they would reflect true inner-and-outer beauty that would then infect more *souls* in our societies (*ripple-effect*) to instigate change. This might be a very naive idea/goal, but if you observe the present world, it is clear that our priorities are off. We are misguided, and this is not serving us. We need to return to basics!

In NH's philosophy, we are mostly focused on our inner cleanliness so that the physical body can function optimally. A person can never look more beautiful than with a healthy glow on the cheeks created by nature herself, and to achieve this, we need to go as deep as to the core of our cells. So, when all conditions are in favor, the body can only give you, besides original health, true:

"Original Beauty"

When it comes to beauty, the skin is, for most people, the most important asset. It is the largest organ that we have, and it is directly exposed to weather elements, beauty products, and other people's view. It has a surface area of between 1.5-2.0 square meters (*16.1-21.5 sq ft.*), so it is quite the organ to deal with. We feel beautiful and "sexy" when we have a fresh radiant look, if it is real or not. It gives confidence to a person and a secure feeling of health and youthfulness. Sometimes these perceptions, on yourself or others, are fake because of the unnatural products that are delicately, or not, smeared on the face and body to achieve that representation of youth. This applying of makeup by our ladies, and also men, is one of the best ways to quickly look "younger" before heading out in public. So logically, it is the most important market for the beauty industry to concentrate on.

Have you ever read, by the way, anything about "urine therapy?" I have met people that use their own urine on their skin and even drink it, and they really swear by its benefits. Through a book, I once learned that cosmetics even have filtered human urine in it, as it was claimed, but that appears to be incorrect. They created a synthetic form of natural occurring *urea* and indeed use that in their products. They learned of the surprising properties of our unique bodily element and so had to copy it as it is tricky to market urine.

The market for beautifying products is larger than huge. These powerful industries are on a continuous mission to find the fountain of youth: the ultimate anti-aging, multi-billion valued cream. Personally, I think if we do find one day this "Holy Grail," it will be through a genetic breakthrough.

We all certainly want to look and feel younger, but to my knowledge, this is the wrong way to achieve this goal. Beauty is created within. It is the result of inner cleanliness. We all know about the unfortunate diminishing elasticity of our skin that is responsible for the aging effect. The skin's collagen level goes down over time, together with decreased blood flow (*remember the effects of processed sugar, salt, fat, smoking, and alcohol that we explored*). These natural aging effects that we all go through happen to us in many different intensities. Some people just look young longer than others as all of us don't have the same genetic disposition, and it does not seem fair. Even so, we can all still have some control over our aging by being aware of the lifestyle we follow.

Be cautious about applying products to your skin, as your skin is an organ. A very sensitive organ that needs, like the insides of your body, a decent amount of love and care. A very important *natural law* is broken when not abiding by one fundamental treatment: that your skin needs to—breathe!

I am fully aware that many people swear by the special treatments they receive at their beauty parlor/spa. I am also sure that they feel that their plastic surgery, botox injections, and laser treatments together with that new expensive cream, keep them looking younger. The caution here is that these are, to my knowledge, temporary fixes. You may look better for some time, but nature has her own way of "payback" when her delicate balance is disturbed. Try your best to minimize any man-made products and treatments.

When it comes to face and body lifts, sometimes there is a need and benefit to have those done, but the often unnatural looking results make it worse. Maybe one day, when we all live cleaner lifestyles that support beautiful aging, we will see no more need to manipulate—nature's design. This brings us to another important statement:

> ***"All processed unnatural products that the skin is exposed to are toxic to your health and beauty"***

This is essential to understand. The average hair, skin, and mouth products are filled with chemicals. These unnatural toxic elements are absorbed, like a sponge, by your delicate skin membranes. Your body then needs to process and remove these toxins from your system to bring back "homeostasis."

I know that it is not easy to avoid using products as we are creatures of habit. This *action* has become a social practice with the help and encouragement of the beauty industry, of course. This applying behavior is similar to the urge to assist the body by taking medicines when not feeling well.

We think that the body needs assistance. Nothing is further from the truth. Then the most important action within NH's philosophy for you to follow is the act of,—doing nothing! Because the body is self-correcting. The clever marketing strategies that exist on all levels of our commercial world would have you believe that the body needs help. Please be aware of this. If you are like most people buying beautifying products, I would suggest to slowly remove them from your life. But, if you still feel that you need to apply, there are many animal-friendly and chemical-free beauty products for you to explore. The inhumane cruelties taking place in beauty laboratories that experiment on innocent creatures are just shocking. Decide to not be a part of this. Please absorb this fact through your "empathetic" skin. You will then feel that this practice is barbaric and unjust.

"Be kind to our loving animals"

But even though the ingredients of beauty products have improved, they are still manufactured in a laboratory. They are impure elements that contain preservatives. These beauty products are not alive! So, then the new "mantra" to follow is:

"We consume alive foods,—and we apply alive foods"

In the world of NH we are constantly focused on the "endogenous" (*internal*) and "exogenous" (*external*) toxins. The influences of the physical world upon our living system are plentiful. Due to the pollution of the air, soil, and water, we are constantly bombarded by toxins. Once you have learned about the many threats that exist upon your health, avoiding these toxins will become a normal part of your life.

People have told me: "Ah, that is crazy, that is no life if you have to constantly watch what you eat and do!" "Not if you choose health," is my usual response. Once you have applied those cleaner choices to your life, they become second nature without a thought. It is all about choice.

What do you choose?

I often wonder how the world and people's health would look like if we never had to deal with the corrupt practices of greedy industries polluting our health and planet. A world without lies and deceit in the processed and chemical-laden food industry. Utopian thoughts come to mind.

Let's have a look now at some of these external toxic products that should be avoided. Please note that we have no separate *transitional* and *cleaner* suggestions in this *step*, as there is only one way to deal with these health violations.

Sunscreen—A major blow to many people's belief system is that sunscreens are dangerous. Like with all other beauty products, they contain an extensive collection of chemicals. Sunscreen's purpose is to block the sun from entering our skin, and that is the idea you might say. But the fact is that the sun "NEEDS" to enter your skin, to keep your vital vitamin D levels up. Sunshine maintains a healthy body as it recharges you naturally. To some extent, it will even nourish you so that you have less need for physical food.

But if you have a sensitive hide, then your exposure to our life-giving rays needs to be build up carefully. We all have been guilty of exposing ourselves to the point of *burning* even to a crisp. And all this suffering for a,—tan. This is not the way to go about it, and when you do insist on frying yourself, well, then, yes, you need to block your sun exposure. But the right course of action is that when you feel that tingling sensation on your skin, to remove yourself, it's that simple. So, the only true sunscreen then for you to use is:

SHADE

We are naked animals by nature. This means that we are designed to be outdoors and unclothed as our total body surface benefits from the exposure to those warm golden rays. Another fact is that we are tropical, or at least, sub-tropical mammals. We need to frolic in the sun. It is our predestined state of happiness. I do agree that we have to be careful with our sun exposure, especially these days. But luckily, we have, to some degree, a defense against too much damage. Our protection is the tanning of the skin. One of the main reasons for dealing with these sun vulnerabilities is because of our over-exposure. Over the ages, we have removed ourselves from the shady jungles where we came from and felt at home (*the chopping down of our green world does not help either*).

When I need to find answers in life concerning diet and lifestyle, I reflect back to our very distant primitive past. Where we lived in our natural habitats of dense green jungles and forests with a moderate to high humidity (*there is no better moisturizer*). We were naturally protected from the sun by the tree canopies, and our exposure was minimum. Just half an hour of soothing sunshine, will already give you health, happiness, nourishment, and vitamin D. So, do not be afraid of it, just be cautious and tan sensibly if you can.

Shampoos and Soaps—When we bathe, one of the first things we do is grab the soap and lather up a fluffy foam to clean our body with, and we cannot imagine not doing this. Remember that these products are also unnatural substances. They often contain cheap foaming agents and perfumes to entice you to keep using them. We have the same truth here as with all beauty products. These soaps are absorbed through your skin and exposed to your delicate system, which needs to spend energy on removing these violations from its tissues.

The purpose of soap is to collect the dirt from your skin, which then washes off, leaving your body squeaky clean with a nice smell. However, that feeling of cleanliness creates a problem for the skin as you have removed all its natural oils. Soaps are mostly too harsh on our delicate hair and body because they create an imbalance on an epidermic level that the body needs to correct again. And the smell of strawberries or flower essence is just a wrong perception. It is a fake fragrance created in a lab. Do you really want to give your skin an artificial feeling of cleanliness and odor? When eating clean, it is enough to rinse with only warm water to remove your excess body odor. But if you continue eating irritating foods, like garlic and onions, that escape through your skin, no soap in the world can truly remove those "pungent" smells.

And when you step out of the shower ready for the world again, I bet that you will go next for your deodorant. Regular products are definitely toxic, so a suggestion is to wash those underarms with warm water more frequently. Or make your own deodorant with coconut and tea tree oil, as they are both strong natural antibacterials.

So, although warm to hot water for your body is usually enough, the exception to the rule is maybe when you worked with grease or paint. Like, when you have been working on your car or been painting the baby room. One can get pretty dirty in either case, so extra help is often needed. In these extreme situations, you will need to use a degreaser. Please find in your local health food store an animal-friendly skin soap (*no petrochemicals*) that you will only use for these challenging cleaning jobs. So that you can get yourself ready on time for your dinner party or maybe a romantic date. Better yet is to use gloves and a coverall.

The same story goes for your hair. Only thorough rinsing is usually sufficient. Hair and scalp need natural oils, so if you have a problem with extremely oily hair and skin, you will need to look at your diet. The same goes for the opposite condition. Remember that the use of toxic table salt creates dry, flaky skin, so you will be helping your scalp and hair by adapting the hygienic rule, "NO salts and spices."

I have not used shampoo for ages (*on the hair that I have left*) as the scalp will self-cleanse and rebalance over time. In some rural areas of Costa Rica, women cannot afford the fancy soaps from the western world (*lucky for them*). They rinse their hair with rainwater captured by a flower in its interior. Oh! You should smell that water, it's incredible. You can also soak flower peddles to create fragrant water that you can use for your body and hair to rinse with. With a little imagination, you can completely change your beauty routine.

Let's not forget that we also need to address all the hair dyes and other chemicals our "hair artists" use in their trade. These are highly toxic as they reportedly have a direct linkage to certain cancers. But I understand that when you see those grey hairs appearing that it is not easy to do. When faced with a decision between your health and your looks, you will need to consult with your doctor (*if he is aware of the dangers*).

Skin Creams—Because we removed our natural oils with the harsh chemical soaps we used, we often need to replace them again. Which is clearly very counterproductive. And as far as the lotions or creams go that give you a moisturized feeling, well, the ingredients there are usually some kind of nasty refined oils from the petrochemical industry. Always read labels and pay attention to what your skin is telling you.

We need to be much kinder to our *natural armor*. So, as I mentioned earlier, the solution here is to use a high water content skin-soothing living food that you actually can eat. I met this lady once who would smear mango peel on her skin. Granted, it is not something you usually observe, and she looked a bit yellow for most of the day. Still, she said that her skin never felt better when she showers it off in the evening. Personally, I use fresh "Aloe Vera" straight from the plant that I apply after some exposure to sunshine or shaving. I also recommend using organic coconut butter or oil, which is very beneficial for most skins. You might already have experienced beauticians using fresh cucumbers or kiwi's on your eyes or avocados. They are catching on, so what is stopping you?

Makeup—These cosmetics sure are tricky because many women would not leave home without it, as already explored. Unfortunately, this grooming habit is very toxic. Research what alternatives you could use, like pomegranate seeds for your lips. When you research the ingredients of cosmetics, one can only become disgusted and appalled!

- Snail mucus (*skin creams*)
- Placenta (*masks and lotions*)
- Whale vomit (*perfumes*)
- Genital secretion (*perfumes*)
- Placenta (*masks and lotions*)
- Crushed bugs (*lipstick*)

And if that is not all, various heavy metals are found in the average makeup line. Metals like lead, cadmium, and arsenic. Needless to say here that these are extremely poisonous. Fortunately, you can find in the health food store natural beauty products that are metal-free and Vegan. However, they still have processed ingredients in them. I would suggest to try these and to minimize cosmetic use as much as possible.

Toothpaste—I already had to "newsflash" you on *page 131* that toothpaste is toxic, and you are better off not using it. One suggestion is to use only warm water with your brush or just rinse your mouth with water/saliva. Then, you can use celery stalks to alkalize your mouth with. Also, garlic and onions are not really covered in this book. Against popular belief, they are toxic to the system, as the body expels these irritants through your skin. We all are familiar with the smells emanating from a person (*skin and breath*) after their garlic meal. If you remove them from your diet, you will prevent many unpleasant mouth and body odors. You could chew on some fresh parsley or mint leaves, which is great for masking odors, but prevention will always be a safer bet. I personally brush only with water, and occasionally, I add some naturally produced sodium bicarbonate. It helps to maintain bright looking teeth (*keep in mind to use it only infrequently as it is mildly abrasive and can damage your enamel*).

Following a cleaner diet, which means no more staining with coffee, tea, red wine, spices, and cigarettes, is all you need to do to support a—beautiful smile.

Shaving Cream—One for both the sexes. It is toxic and needs to be avoided. The best alternative here is aloe vera, avocado, or coconut oil. You can buy aloe leaves at the health food store. Or because this succulent (*stores water in its leaves*) grows easily in many climates, grow it yourself for easy availability and freshest source. Smear it on your skin before/after shaving or bedtime. It takes a bit of getting used to as it is soo slimy, but nature really has no better moisturizer than this clear gooey. **Tip**: scoop/scrape it out of the leaves, blend it up with lemon juice (*preservative*), avocado, and/or coconut oil and store in a jar, and keep in your fridge.

Let's look now at a few everyday cheap household products that I urge you to remove from your immediate environment. These products can be replaced with little effort.

Dish Washing Liquid—This stuff is only needed when you have greasy pots and pans to deal with, and with my suggested diet changes, you will have no more of those. Not to sound too paranoid, but when using this toxic stuff found on every supermarket shelf in vibrant neon colors, it will leave a film of residue behind on your plate or bowl that will come off into your food when eaten from or pots when cooked in. All these chemicals build up in your system, do not forget. There are healthier soap alternatives, but rinsing with a sponge and hot water will do the trick when eating clean. Like with showering, you can keep some natural soap on hand for when you have a more tasking dishwashing job to do.

Cleaning Products—They are used for various cleaning jobs around the house, and each kind has its own purpose. Guaranteed that you will find in every household at least five different cleaning agents, if not more, under the sink. The chemical attack on your direct health and the environment, which is also a part of you, is immense. Please make a serious effort to find replacements for these evils. As I already mentioned, natural dishwashing liquid can already cover many greasy tasks. Then, we have natural lemon for some particular cleansing and maybe some bleaching jobs. We have baking soda that can also cover many challenges. It only needs a scrubbing brush and maybe vinegar as its sidekick to remove odors and stains. Question all the products you have in your cabinets and look for another way to deal with the problem. Your health will be a reflection of this decision.

Air Fresheners—I have been into a house once that had electric air fresheners in practically every room. I remember thinking: "What do they have to hide?" As you can imagine, these products are plainly said, "poison," and only mask the problem. It is often the furniture's fabric, nylon carpets or unnatural (*cheap*) materials used in the house's construction that will produce a smell when it is damp. Try to find these culprits and replace them when you can with more natural material. The best defense is exactly the same as with the body. When the underlying cause is removed, bad odors will disappear. Also, watch out for those scented garbage bags!

This same philosophy goes for the bathroom. I dated a girl once who always made me laugh. She walked into the toilet one time, and she immediately sprayed this air freshener before anything else. When I asked her why she does that, she replied: "Why should I sit in my own bad smells?" To me, that was very funny, but these cans of fake fragrances are the worst you can sit in or walk into. Open a window or light a match, which is an old trick, but leave those sprays out of your life. Or you could, as I keep on pushing, finally wave those offensive smells goodbye by eating more healthy and clean, and so create a friendlier stomach content. The rest of your household will thank you.

Gas and Poo

The collection and disposal of our own body's waste, is of great importance. As a matter of fact, our trash collection and the disposing and/or burning it on landfills placed in our beautiful pure nature stinking up the air and polluting the groundwater, is a direct correlation to health or disease for the environment, if you understand what I mean with this.

We often crack practical jokes about passing gas in movies and social circles, and admittedly those can be really funny. But the seriousness of it is never really recognized. Many reasons exist for passing gas, and more often than not, it is a sign of trouble in your bowel machine. To keep this simple, when you pass gas with a real offending odor, there is trouble, and your diet and/or food-combining practice needs to be corrected (*see other chapters in this book*). Gas can/will also be created when eating high fiber foods, like apples, pears, grapes, etc., (*the bacteria in the colon produces gas as a byproduct from digesting fiber*). When it does not come with bad odor this effect is nothing to worry about.

We also breathe wrong or eat too hastily, which will result in the swallowing of air that needs to come out eventually. Focused breathing techniques exist that you can learn, and a relaxed meal with proper chewing is the best practice.

And to talk about "poo." Many jokes there too, and besides us all being grossed out about this hopefully daily elimination process, we hardly ever give it any real thought. Constipation is a huge problem in our western world, and the addictive use of laxatives to solve it creates even more issues (*see page 202*). If you do not sit at least once a day on your *white throne*, there is a cry for change. Technically, there should be a movement after each 12-hour digestion cycle. So, two a day, when you ate easy digestible natural foods with tons of fiber (*when you eat real nutritional foods, you will do better with only two meals a day*). And when one, two, or more days are skipped, waste is lingering and toxifying your system. A statement I found once sums this all up beautifully:

"We have big hospitals and small stools!"

When your feces reek profusely, you are abusing your system and need to fix what is broken. Also, make sure you maintain a bulky dark or greenish stool color (*indicates much green in your diet*), as a bleak skimpy one is a sign of a poor diet, with no fiber and greens. Then a final hint that your poo machine needs oiling is the quick or slow passage. As you have learned in this book, digestion and your waste removal needs to happen fast. When on your porcelain throne, reading a whole newspaper, having to force the exit, and nothing to show in the end, then you need to know that there is trouble on the horizon.

Another fact is that if we all would eat cleaner, we could save the planet by not chopping down our trees! Using toilet paper is not really needed when you care for your bowel system. So, pay attention to your "poo and gas" as they play an essential part in your well-being.

Air—There is definitely nothing worse than breathing stale air, so make sure that you keep your house aired. I understand that we cannot all live in the pure mountain air of the Swiss Alps, but try the best you can to keep your house smelling fresh and ventilated. You could purchase an "air ionizer" that removes toxic particles from the air. But they seem to be a bit unreliable in doing what they claim, so look into this if you have no other choice because opening your window will only invite car or factory pollution in (*moving is another option*). Specific plants in the house, especially in your bedroom, can help as well as they produce oxygen. The body is cleansing itself during the night, and you will awaken more invigorated.

Pets—Where would we be without our pets? You just have to love them. Animals do better in a cleaner environment as well, so give them what you are giving yourself. Keep their sleeping quarters clean and fresh, including their food and water. A house can quickly reek of your animals if they are not well taken care of. Bathe your loving pets in warm water. If you have to use a product, use one that will not irritate their delicate skin. Your pet's health also benefits from a raw natural diet, so research what this is. We always had big dogs when I grew up, and I remember that two of them got cancer and had to be put down. The reason, we fed them mostly our cooked food scraps. Also, check the quality of your pet's dry food before buying! When a particular "pet candy" or toy in a store looks cute and can be nibbled on for fun does not mean you should buy it. Your pet should not eat any artificial food as they are also very prone to imbalances. You will notice improvements when given a more natural lifestyle.

As a last suggestion, please do not adopt any animals not suited for house-living, just stick to the domesticated ones.

When a client asks me to come over and suggest changes in their home, I am always amazed at what needs to be done. The list is pretty much the same every time, as people have routinely the same dangerous products around the house. I get real satisfaction from cleaning up a home. It feels almost like exorcising a house of,—"bad spirits" (*if you believe in them*).

Radiation—And talking about something that is there, but you cannot see it. We have another invisible danger to your health, called WiFi! It goes hand in hand with all the other electromagnetic radiation around the house! Do the needed research to have peace of mind. The media still tells us that it is not hazardous to our health, but please ignore that.

Cellphone companies are the worst when it comes to hiding factual research from the public eye. Smartphones/speakers, computers, and tablets all represent a risk. Now they are rolling out 5G, and it needs to be told that it is dangerous. Try to make at least your bedroom WiFi proof for a deep solid sleep without radiation frying your brain all night long (*you can cover the walls and ceiling with special material*).

We could easily come up with more hazardous unhealthy products/practices around the house, there is plenty more, but I'll stop here as I am sure that you got the message.

The Final Curtain

We have come to the last pages of this "self-help" book, and I hope you had as much fun reading it as I enjoyed writing this for you. In this small book, I have shared the most important points/steps to help you on your way to a cleaner, happier, and healthier life. Allow yourself this *empowerment* that lets you control your own health fate. Eliminate disease from your life, and make sure that from now on, you will only need to:

"Go and see your doctor when HE is not feeling well"

As you have learned, disease is an unnatural state of being that does not serve you in any way. Recognize that you and your loved ones are being conditioned to adopt a lifestyle that suits the large money-making corporations. A certain degree of "wakening up" is needed here. I do not know about you, but I feel liberated when I can express my own views. When I can live in a way that I have learned is healthier for me, instead of accepting the corrupt spoon-fed information stream diminishing our personal powers. Brave your beliefs and be your own *Self*, as we are all unique in the eyes of nature.

What is the point of it all when your personal path in life is hindered or cut short because of some dreaded illness or early death? That is no fun! We need to reevaluate what matters.

This is what I would like to leave you with. A sense of the magnificence and mysticism that surrounds our lives. We are soo insignificantly small in the grandness of the Universe, but yet we are an intricate part of this immensity. Never take life and your health for granted. Experience every momentous moment in this human game called—evolution.

For now, we need to make a conscious effort to improve our health and quality of life. For yourself, your fellow man across the land, and our,—Mother Earth.

Because we are all ONE!

* * * * * *

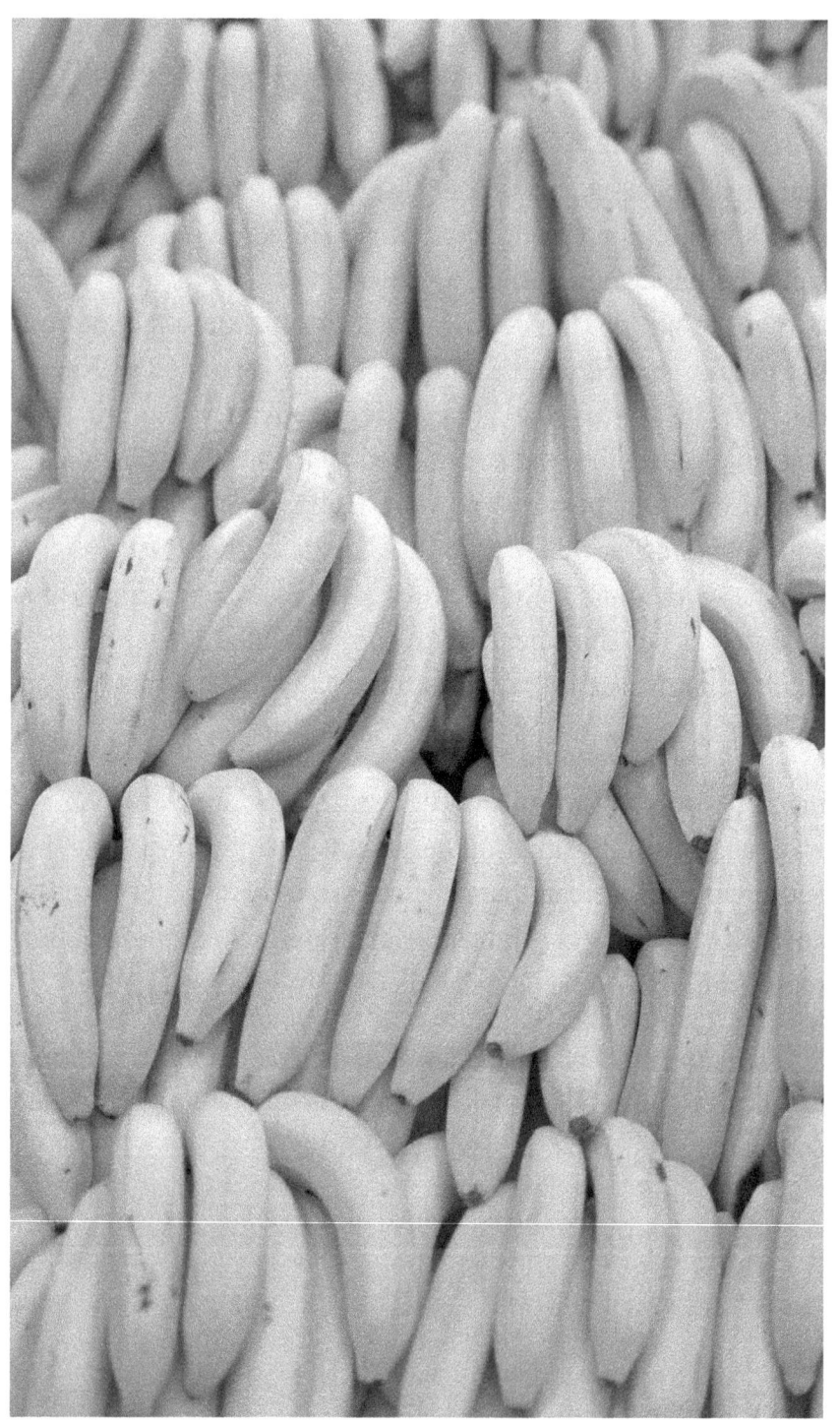

YOUR NEW BEST FRIENDS

And how could I leave you without introducing you to my best friends that I certainly hope will become yours as well. You are already acquainted with these companions as you have seen them around. And most likely had the pleasure of having them in your kitchen or, hopefully, on your plate.

The world is stocked with a wide variety of juicy fruits of all shapes, colors, and tastes. I have been to countries where they had fruit that could have come straight from the planet "Pandora" (*Avatar movie*). So utterly weird and unknown to most people, including myself. But even the familiar fruits that we consume have many different varieties, like the mango and banana. It is just incredible that there are over a thousand assorted banana species and roughly around four hundred other kinds of mango delights.

So, I am saying here that there is no chance you ever get bored with fruits. I read a business article from Wallmart once, the biggest supermarket chain in the world, what their biggest selling individual item is. To many peoples shocking surprise, it is the. . .♪drum roll♪. . ."banana!" This surely tells us something. They are truly the king of fruits. They have all you need under one yellow jacket, so I hope you enjoy them because they are the first on my best friends list.

Bananas—They are the fruits designed for the human race. It is a very ancient fruit and actually a perennial herb, so they do not grow on a tree. They are available all year round, which is important when adopting a more fruit-based diet. They are extremely satisfying and loaded with responsible nutrition. Furthermore, the whole essential "amino acids" family is on board, so a great usable source of protein. The high water density and sugar content guarantee a healthy hydration level and your sweet tooth fix. Personally, I could not follow the *raw food diet* without bananas. Enjoy them whole or in a smoothie. They satiate me the best.

Avocado—High water content, fiber, predigested enzymes, minerals, vitamins, friendly fat, and protein content are all the personal traits of this amigo. People worry about the fat, but it is a "monounsaturated" fatty acid, so better to digest, and heart friendlier than animal fat. It is also a great replacement for butter (*which you now not consume any more of course*)

Many varieties exist, but the Haas is the most commercial one we know. This creamy friend is genuinely one of the best nutritious foods. Eat an avocado with your evening meal when you have a strenuous next day ahead, like an intense yoga class or 10 km run. It never fails for me when working out in the gym, as I feel strong and supported for endurance.

Dates—There are around 150 types of dates. For me, I got stuck with the Medjools. It was love at first bite. So moist and sweet, and guaranteed to satisfy your cravings for sugar. This natural candy can be enjoyed without any guilty thoughts. You can use them in raw desserts, in smoothies, or eaten by themselves as they digest quickly when properly combined. These highly nutritious goodies are best consumed organic because then they can be called "One of the most nutritious foods on the planet!"

These are the foods I consume most in the winter (*when I am not in the tropics*). When it comes to the summer, I have a whole lotta more friends to play with. I will go crazy over watermelon, kiwi's, mangoes, apples, pears, grapes, oranges, any type I can get my hands on really. Our natural instincts will guide us to eat more fruits when it is hot. As we are then "catapulted" back to our primal habitat of the jungle where we technically belong. Our bodies will tell us to hydrate and nourish, so that we will be able to "thrive" instead of just survive, and so taking care of our amazing—vehicle.

A Fruit Debate

A question that many people, including health professionals, have is, "Should we eat the fruits that are technically out of season?" With our present-day fast international transport network, a person can eat tropical mangoes for breakfast from the other side of the planet. The argument is that we should only eat the goodness of the Earth that is in season locally.

The "carbon footprint" the world is worrying about tells us that we are indeed dealing with a problematic system (*food, people, and mail transport*). But one could argue that if all our means of transportation were electric, thus, no pollution attached to the shipping of tropical delights, it would become an acceptable trade-off. But some people just feel that it is unnatural to eat bananas, kiwi's, coconuts, and papayas, for sale in the supermarket in the midst of winter in the west.

My personal view is that although I agree with the issues of moving tropical fruits all over the planet, as it stresses our environment, the consumption of fruit from another season is a good thing. Don't forget that we are tropical, or at least sub-tropical animals, and we are not supposed to live in the colder regions of our world. We need to live in the parts where our fruits grow pretty much all year round. Cold and arctic climates are unnatural and unhealthy, despite the many thousands of years that some cultures have survived there (*the colder it gets where you are, the more unhealthy it is*). Even living in a four-season region is not ideal. Let's recap what we need for radiant health:

- ✔ Sunlight for warmth & Vit. D (*be as naked as possible*)
- ✔ Clear blue skies for eye health (*total light spectrum*)
- ✔ Fresh warm air (*breathing cold air is not natural*)
- ✔ Structured water (*from our fruit sources*)
- ✔ Outdoor living for sanity (*not confined indoors*)
- ✔ Year-round gardening (*for continuous fresh food*)

To sum it up. If a region of the world only produces delicious fruit and greens three months out of the year, like strawberries, apples, pears, spinach, lettuce, celery, and rely the remaining months on greenhouses and imports, we are not really supposed to live there. Technically, we would then be forced to seek other food sources, like local animals, root vegetables, and other cold season foods that grow in the cold darkness of the soil. Our true food sources, nourished by the sun's healing rays, cannot grow year-round and therefore are absent from our diet (*we can survive, but not thrive!*).

So, we all move to the sub/tropics or be grateful for our transportation system. I hope that mankind will learn one day that tropical fruits are our best source of nutrition, and we then start growing it everywhere where possible. But until that day, I would say: "Enjoy your fruits wherever you are as nothing is perfect and your health is important." Thankfully, we are now heading for a cleaner carbon-free transportation system (*electric planes, ships, and cars*) so that one day in a more Utopian world, we can really enjoy our fruits guilt-free!

* * * * * *

QUESTIONS & ANSWERS

In this last segment of the book, we will address some of the frequent questions I receive from curious and confused people about certain aspects of health. Wellness seekers approach me with these important inquiries as they feel that many different opinions and philosophies exist in the realms of health these days, and they are right. These confusions exist because of the misdirections of the "media world," financed by the food corporations! Plus, we also have too many "self-proclaimed" health experts that *fuel* the confusion to sell a book or to promote a food product (*they're funded by businesses*). It is complicated to differentiate the truths from the "non-sense!"

As I suggested early in the book, you need to research these confusing irregularities yourself when looking to find an answer. For me, the most powerful "mind opener" and so tactic that I use to find the answer (*as I explained before*) is the logical approach of observing nature. Then, to ask myself: "What makes the most sense?" Of course, this is not always a 100% foolproof method in finding the complete truth of whatever concerns you, but it is a start.

For example, when it comes to food, it is a lot faster to rule out the foods that are part of our kitchen today, but that never existed before in nature. Like donuts, pies, pizza, cornflakes, and spaghetti, to name a few *unnatural* food items. Then, the microwaving of food, GMOs, laser, hair dyeing, botox and vaccine injecting, smartphones EM radiation, etc., which are all mankind's so-called advancements. By: "never existed before," I mean that these foods, technologies, and practices were never a part of our "natural world." And never can be! Thus, they are considered a danger to our natural health.

Always be aware that many adopted practices, behaviors, and foods have become inherently normal over time. To read that somebody, like me, dismisses these ain't always easy, so give it some thought and time. Okay, .. let's get to it.

How come that I keep on reading many health articles claiming that a cup of coffee or wine is good for me, as research was conducted on this?

Understand that these particular magazine/Internet/newspaper articles are financed by the producers and/or investors of these products to keep the misinformation alive that they are good for you. Know that these companies do not care about your health. They are ruthless and will stop at nothing to make a trusted believer out of you. They need money-making consumers. They fund these so-called respectable researchers or lab people for large sums of money to make these false health claims. I have often even suspected that these immoral individuals do not even exist in real life.

I am so confused as to what to believe about vaccinations. Our government has our best intentions in mind, no? How can you say that we should stay away from them? We did eradicate polio, didn't we? So, what is your opinion?

This is a tricky one, and a pet project to me. Vaccinations are utterly and unarguably TOXIC to you. They contain many dangerous poisons, like neurotoxic mercury (thimerosal), aluminum, formaldehyde, and aborted human fetal tissue, of all ingredients! Presently, we have a solid belief in place that vaccines are safe and protect us from disease which is, of course, financed by the "medical machine." Governments and the CDC *(Center for Disease Control)* are in cahoots with each other, make no mistake about it. Mercury, e.g., is one of the most toxic elements in existence! So how can anyone claim then that vaccinations are safe to be injected into a person's body, even as young as babies? The propaganda is based on the message of fear: "Protect yourself and your family from disease!" How is the injecting with "toxic filth" going to prevent you from sickness or death from a virus or bacteria? The science behind it is clearly to create a so-called boosted *defense* system by introducing an "enemy" to your immune arsenal, and so creating antibodies.

This is a good one, I'll give them that. Interestingly, this is similar to how nature does it. Still, it is just NOT the natural way to strengthen the immune system with injecting toxins. Here we see mankind's arrogance and greed hard at work to find a way to cash in on natures, in their eyes, imperfect design. This practice is ludicrous and even criminal.

Without a doubt, our defense system has grown weak over time because of our disconnection and disruption of nature. Several causes are chemical pollution, genetic manipulations, water treatments, processed foods, and living in concrete jungles. Also, our cleanliness phobias (*instigated by the businesses that sell cleaning products*) have alienated us from the good bacteria. Trust that a balanced alkaline system that you are working on now will give you a healthy army of microbes that will protect you from disease.

One aspect of life that many forget is the natural system in place that keeps the populations down. In the animal kingdom "The law of the jungle," means that the weakest will perish to disease or will get eaten by a predator. As insensitive this may sound, we are maybe not meant to develop, to some extent, all these toxic medications and treatments to save lives.

So, because of their tactic of fear, we are easily gripped by this *brainwashing,* and we'll do anything to help ourselves and our loved ones by adhering to these false claims. We all want to keep our families safe and healthy, that is our human nature, but at what cost? Think about it . . . they are preying on the uninformed and billions are made. Like when winter is upon us and the "flu weapon" is being used. Or when a new "virus" breaks out (*we are all very familiar with this scenario now*) and we are told to get a shot (*Corona vaccinations are up next*). I hope that you have learned here that this does not sit right. The latest now is that even carcinogenic *Glyphosate* (*Roundup, Monsanto-Bayer*) is found in many vaccines.

And what about "polio?" Interestingly, this is often the first example a person uses to make skeptics against vaccines come to reason. They feel that the eradication of this disease laid the groundwork for progressive medicine and future cures. The Salk vaccine (*named after the researcher Jonas Salk, who produced the first polio vaccine*) is believed by the world to have saved us, but did it? The answer to that is a book upon itself, but this is what I have learned:

"Polio wasn't vanquished,—it was redefined"

Before the polio injection was even declared safe (*1955*), it was first tested on about a million children (*guinea pigs*). After the first inoculations, the numbers of polio cases in the late 50s did indeed start to go down. But this was not because of the effectiveness of this "miracle medicine." What was conveniently omitted from this heroic story why numbers went down was not "medical," but rather "administrative."

Curiously, the history records show us that the numbers were already going down even before the first toxic dose was introduced to a child, so something else was going on. To save face and public scrutiny and to also meet their project objectives, the US government "redefined polio." They altered the symptoms and definitions of the polio condition. By doing this, the disease started to be diagnosed by other names, and so fewer numbers of actual polio cases were reported. So in a sense, the polio symptoms got "diluted" in the medical system. Plus, it has never been really proven that vaccines actually do work. There is plenty we can do naturally to protect ourselves from disease. I believe that the improvement in all areas of hygiene has contributed to better health for all. Like, improving personal and public sanitary conditions and separating human living situations from animal stock. Also, the eradicating of pests, like cockroaches, rats, mice, and fleas, contributed to public health (*many of these are now forced underground into the sewer system*).

The debates around vaccines are on-going and will never cease. The "Pro-Vaccine" and "Anti-Vaccine" proponents will continue to advocate its safety and its dangers. When you read the history of vaccines introduced somewhere in the 19th Century, you learn about the supposedly lifesaving tales of vaccines through various diseases and epidemics. But also about the early protests from the general public and the unnecessary deaths through vaccinations.

My thoughts on this topic are in no way fully expressed, but I know instinctively that injecting with a toxic man-made concoction is not the answer, but a lifestyle change is.

I urge you to watch a fascinating but very controversial documentary called "Vaxxed" *(and Vaxxed II)*. "They" have tried to ban its showings in 2016 and 2019 as the truths in these films will shock you.—"It will wake you up!"

What do you think about the use of superfoods, like chlorella, maca, wheatgrass, and spirulina?

Powdered superfoods are an expensive way to supplement a bad diet and lifestyle. They are not *whole* as a food. They are heated and dried to make a powder that adds to liquids or foods for extra vitamin/nutrient density. But, even so, I cannot completely brush them aside because when a person, for whatever reason, has no access to fresh produce, one needs to supplement until the situation changes.

If you feel that you need to have a powdered supplement, you could then work with a dehydrator machine (*or sunshine*) to dry the *wheatgrass* or fresh *spirulina* yourself and then blend them into a powder. This way, you know at least that it is *raw*. But still, I have to finish again with my best advice:

"Eat whole—Eat fresh!"

By eating *alive foods*, you will be consuming superfoods. Don't buy too quickly into the craze of this growing market. It is just another expensive convenience food that you can do without when having access to fresh food. Keep it simple!

How much fruit and vegetables does a person have to eat to be able to feel satiated? I cannot imagine eating lots of these in one sitting. Is there another way to increase my health still by eating some cooked foods? It seems strict.

I always reply by saying that my suggestions and good advice are not really strict, but,—nature is. I am only the messenger. Nature does not have the deliberate intention to be this severe, but our natural system of life demands to be governed by laws,—biochemical laws. When you are slowly increasing your natural food intake, you will become amazed about how you start to feel more satiated as you are giving yourself real nutrition. But some time to adjust is needed here.

"We eat too much, too often, and too poorly," I always say. The body gets stuck in a perpetual cycle of low nutrition and hunger. Your stomach is a muscle, and when it becomes "trained" to handle more food, it will become much easier to consume your required amount of natural goodness to feel full. If you presently eat two apples and cannot eat more, but feel hungry again in an hour, you still have some *expanding* to do before only fruit can sustain you, so,—patience.

When we lived in the era of foraging from the land, before fire and hunting tools, we needed to sustain ourselves by consuming what was found. It seems plausible to assume that our ancestors were scouring daily their habitats for food. They would move in groups, maybe even making camp on the spot where foods were found. And when finding edible grasses, nuts, raw eggs, fruits, he/she or they would eat until satiated. (*note that the fruits and vegetables from back then cannot be compared with what we have in the supermarket today*).

Life is a heck of a lot easier when you do not have to go to work and turn your endless *hamster wheel* of responsibilities. I imagine that back then, there was nothing else to do than eat, sleep, defecate, and procreate (*maybe an occasional cave painting?*). Primitive man's pooping was also an essential part of the life-cycle, as fruit seeds were unknowingly, like all animals did, planted to secure future food sources.

So, they ate until they moved on as they ran out of food or other reason. But if simple prehuman life was anything as the historians think it was, those folks had more than enough foods to eat (*even with plenty of animal competition*). Those dense jungles and forests had everything growing wild and uninhibited. Natures shelves were/are always stocked if we let it do its thing. It was/is truly a magical fruitful system.

So, to answer the last part. To achieve better health, one would become at least a beautiful Vegan that cooks some foods (*steam as much as possible*) but incorporates as much fresh as he/she can. This diet will become even more healthy when also avoiding wheat, salt, alcohol, you know, as you just read this book. Once you set your goal, you muster up some solid discipline and just "GO" for it. Many will have moments of doubt but just allow your new life to—unfold.

I read that too much fruit is not good for you as all the sugar creates an acid body. What is your take on that?

"Metabolism is insanely complicated!" Ever since it was hypothesized that our foods PH value when consumed affects our health, there have been endless views on what specific digested foods are then "alkaline" or "acid" forming (*much skepticism exists in the medical research industry for this theory*). The reason why it is all so complicated is because certain initial acid reactions of the body can result in an alkaline system like breathing or exercising, to name two.

Many scientific observations that were used to determine what foods create what type of "Hydrogen Ion Activity" in our system was incorrectly performed by burning the food. Then they measured the acid/alkaline ash that resulted. But you cannot compare the burning of whole undigested foods with the end effect of "metabolized" foods (*after the food has been assimilated and digested by our biochemical system*).

Time and time again, it has been proven that vegetables and fruits produce real health. Digesting animal products present challenges and create an *acid* system. And to answer the question, yes! It is true that fruits are slightly acidic because of the sugar, and many so-called experts use that fact as a reason to have you steer away from our natural delights. But the honest truth is that when eating fruit, you are also taking in plenty of alkalizing minerals, like potassium, calcium, and magnesium, that help your body neutralize that acid sugar and leave you with a clean *alkaline* system. So, go ahead and eat your fruits to your heart's content. And if you really want to play it safe, you can eat greens with your fruits or add them to your smoothie,—yummy!

What is the difference between glycemic index and load?

People aware of the "Glycemic Index" list usually are not informed about the "Glycemic Load." The index lists all the foods that the average consumer buys and its sugar content. It is this nutritional database that creates the most hype and misinformation. The GI list tells you how quickly a food gives up its "carbohydrate molecule" and raises your blood sugar. Many unaware shoppers are told by the "general health media" to avoid the high sugar foods there mentioned, especially the "diabetics" (*you'll never read about a high-fat diet being the true cause of diabetes!*). And, of course, this list shows fruits high sugar content (*as it is our fuel*). But only the informed consumer (*that is you now*) will understand how it all works and the beneficial impact of fruits on your system.

So, when we focus on the importance of sugar content, we see a totally different picture. Besides the essential need for sugar, of equal importance is how the body handles this sugar. We know that we cannot over-stress the pancreas too much and so we need to make sure that our fuel is released slowly into our system. Knowing this truth, we then eat whole fruit sources because of high water and fiber content. This way, we secure a slow release of "energy units" into the bloodstream. And this is the glycemic load. The GL list lets us know the "impact" the food has on our blood sugar. A fruit may have a high GI number, but its GL is usually medium to very low. So, there is nothing to worry about. Just keep on eating whole fruits, greens, little fat, combine properly, practice sequential eating, and exercise regularly. You will be consciously controlling your *sugar spikes* by giving your pancreas a steady natural workout.

How can I adopt a fruit diet when I do not like sweets, but prefer salty?

This can be a tricky one. I understand that many people do not have a sweet tooth, but what is that? As I once was a professional candy eater, I can truly claim that although many fruits are classified as a sweet food, they are not really when compared to pure processed sugar found in sweets and desserts. But even when you are not attracted to sweets, fruit is still a recommended food source that you need for better health. Usually, taste buds have become corrupted over time (*inherited or created*) and now have a set liking for salt.

To remind you again, whatever food you eat, the body will turn it into "glucose," your natural fuel. It will not convert it into salt as your gas! It is sugar you survive on, as your muscles and brain need it (*fat and protein can also be converted into glucose energy, but the main source is always carbohydrates*). Let's not forget that we have more than enough options when it comes to fruits. Many are acid or sub-acid, so less sweet, and you could enjoy those with salad greens, to alleviate the little sweetness. When I eat a large green salad with four sliced apples (*sub-acid*), I am happy and satiated. Don't forget, when you crave salt, your system is out of sync as you are probably consuming too much processed salts. Your body is caught in a loop of poor "natural sodium" intake and excessive "sodium chloride." Even if you prefer a bowl of greens with sprouted lentils to a bowl of fruit, give yourself, and so your body, time to adjust. We are creatures of habit and addiction, but when somebody passionately wants to change their health around, the eating of delicious fruit should not be a problem.

I read that fasting is healthy for you. Is this true, it is not dangerous as most doctors claim?

What is a health book without the topic of "fasting?" I am happy that fasting is becoming a more accepted practice now even though it has been around for thousands of years. An uninformed MD will still tell you that it is dangerous to abstain from eating. But this is nonsense, as the countless beneficial reports of people tell us the opposite. Like many important topics concerning health, this one as well deserves a book by itself, so I will only highlight the most important aspects. I can always be contacted for consulting.

First, it is not some kind of miraculous cure for all. Not even everybody notices improvements in their health or a reversal of their chronic condition during or after a fast. But rest assured that you will always reap the benefits. Only the body knows what needs to be done and what is a priority!

A lot of our natural energy gets spent on our digestive process. When no food is consumed, the body has time, and energy, to spend on other important tasks, like deep tissue cleansing. During a fast, one still drinks pure water to help the process and to stay hydrated. One can also do a "juice fast," so only fruit juices are taken in. Beneficial for sure, but a deep cleansing is not achieved as this is still eating. All bodily processes need energy! When the body is constantly drained of this resource through wrong diet, poor sleep, stress load, etc., it will never have the opportunity to reset and detoxify properly which has become soo important in our fast lives. You must admit that the thought of your body cleansing the "nooks and crannies" of your body, like spring cleaning your house, sounds pretty rewarding.

The human body can survive (*safely*) without food for up to 30 days. But Dr. Herbert Shelton, the founding father of NH, supported people who did much longer fasts, even up to 90 days. My recommendation is always that when planning a fast for over two weeks (*one week if the faster has a medical condition*), a licensed physician should be present. Fasting once or twice a year should be a routine in everybody's life so that we can clean and reset our systems.

Talking about fasting, an alarming trend has resurfaced or is being reinvented, called "dry fasting." This is becoming a thing now, and it worries me. A person will, besides food, also not take in any liquids for a period of time. The benefits are claimed to be an improved immune system, lower blood pressure, and better glucose levels. I honestly did not give this topic much research because, to me, it is clear. Even though it has been practiced by many cultures and religious traditions throughout history, it comes with safety instructions.

We are water and need it daily to detox and function, so frankly, it is "dangerous!" The folks that started this trend or are sprouting from this ancient practice to sell a book and get clicks need to be careful with these claims. Food fasting is a lot safer and has true benefits, so I would stick with that to assist the body (*the body, as I claim in this book, does not need help, not even fasting, when one follows a clean lifestyle as I recommend*). A very well known action actor told in an interview that when he has a scene coming up where he needs to flex his muscles and show off his many months in the gym, does a three day dry fast because it will make his skin paper-thin and so defining his physique even more. Crazy world!

I am worried about "Genetically Modified" foods. What are the real dangers, and can eating organic protect us?

It is something I worry about as well. Our world has gone mad! Profit and greed are now the world's languages, and when you try to speak a different tongue, you get smothered. Thankfully, people are awakening and start to grow their own foods or buy organic. The need in the last three decades for organic produce has steadily increased, and we all need to support these farmers the best we can.

But we are not yet out of harm's way. Much corruption exists in the organic world as well, even within the food regulating bodies, like the FDA or USDA. Many farmers are up against the wall as they are dealing with powerful and heinous forces. Take Monsanto and Bayer, e.g. (*now merged*), one of the world's most corrupt and evil companies. They continue to poison our planet and, despite all of their lawsuits, are still getting away with environmental destruction. Their GMO foods/seeds contaminate the healthy organic field crops and destroy our hard-working farmer's incomes with their patented *monopoly seeds*. Their *golden goose* product called "Roundup" continues to pollute our groundwater and soil.

But without a doubt, buying organic is still your best option in this perplexity, and from a reputable farmer. Never stop asking questions concerning the water being used, farming methods, fertilizers, or even what the farmer believes and eats him/herself. It is one thing to grow organic to fill a demand, but it is another to farm with firm belief and passion. You, the consumer, still has the power to keep these food producers honest and on their toes. But at the end of the day, you can only trust the Earthly delights you grow yourself.

So, the battle for our health continues. Never hesitate to sign a petition or participate in a peaceful protest to enforce control against these corrupt companies. Staying vigilant is our best—defense!

How do you get enough B12 on a Vegan diet?

Funny enough, this question led me to the path that I am presently on. I once visited a girl, back in 1992, I really liked (*I was a virgin Vegan, so knew not much about it, yet*) and while making lunch, she asked me how do I get enough B12. It totally panicked me that I did not know anything about it and made up an answer to appear knowledgeable. After that embarrassment, I began learning all about healthy living.

B12 is that vital element that we need for daily growth, maintenance, creation of blood, DNA regulation, and very importantly, our nervous system. The amount that we need is minimal but extremely essential. I always hoped that the whole issue around this vitamin was as simple as eating organic fruits and veggies to guarantee your adequate daily intake. Unfortunately, that scenario was wishful thinking. This water-soluble vitamin is very tricky and controversial. It has a long list of ill-conditions up its sleeve that you can fall victim to if you become depleted. Its availability depends mostly on our digestion (*bacteria flora*) and the *soil* that grows our natural foods. The regular health info that you find on the web, or when you talk to a regular MD, is that you have to eat animal products to get it,—case closed! But there is more to it, as you will see.

You can indeed obtain valuable B12 from animals and their byproducts, but interestingly, meat-eaters are also at risk for not getting sufficient levels, so, "That kite is not gonna fly." So, we have together with the soil and the bacteria in our gut these sources to rely on. But still, neither one of these can secure an actual uptake and its usability. There have been plenty of cases where deficient people were injected with B12 over some time but to no avail.

This topic also deserves its own book, but I will share the most essential points that will help you on your way if you just became or are already a Vegan for some years. To me, it is very important that we clarify this and put you at ease.

As the research shows, it all comes down to our bacteria. These little helpers are part of our foundation for healthy living. And as bacteria phobic many people are, you need them. When using the method of logical reasoning, you can only conclude that nature must have, in its perfect design, also a solution for B12. There were no supplements and injections available before the 1950s, and all the way back to our first days on the planet. Otherwise, people would have massively died of B12 deficiencies, like "pernicious anemia," and nerve damage over all those millennia.

Let's do some more logical reasoning. There has to be a way to get it in our original human diet besides animal flesh. Again, we are biologically not designed to consume it. Even once upon a time, we did not eat flesh at all (*I hope that I managed to convince you of this?*). Several important points that need to be thrown into this quest are:

- A) Our lifestyles have become too clean.
- B) We are drugged up (*pharmaceuticals*) and live stressful lives (*destroys intestinal bacteria flora*).
- C) We consume poor nutritious foods.
- D) The soil is polluted and so of bad quality.
- E) We have disconnected ourselves from nature.

Basically, we are summing up the same causes that we find in this book for destroying our "Original Health!"

> *"Remember, when you pollute the soil, you are polluting your health"*

A farmer that uses natural feed for its animals and let it graze on green grass and does not "pump" it full of chemicals would be raising a farm creature entirely toxin-free. Then, this animal's organic manure can be used to fertilize our fresh crops to promote healthy bacteria growth in the soil (*the soil needs to contain "cobalt"*). The bacteria colonies feast on the decaying organic matter and excrete complex nutrients, like B12, to be taken up by the plant or remain in the soil. Animals get their B12 from grazing and it is produced in their gut. So, when we harvest our crops and then would not be too fussy about washing and scrubbing these foods squeaky clean, they could supply us with valuable B12 on a daily basis. This is how it is designed as I tried to make evident in this book:

> *"To absorb our nutrients and vitamins through our environment"*

As I explained, we need to get our hands dirty at times (*leave your garden gloves behind next time when planting those Begonias*). Or roll a bit in the mud so now and then if you can, "fun," but not for everybody. The point I am making here is that we are jeopardizing our precious health by destroying our important *link* with nature by living too wrong, too clean, and too distant.

Furthermore, we need to maintain a healthy balance within. We have to support a thriving bacteria flora that possibly could supply us with that essential vitamin we are discussing here. And if you consider that our stomach cells actually secrete "Intrinsic Factor" that helps the body to absorb B12, it seems clear that we need to respect the workings of the stomach and maintain a balance there at all costs. It is said over and over again, that "True health starts in the gut!" In the Natural Hygiene philosophy, it is stated that naturally a B12 deficiency should not exist:

> "To secure co-enzymes of B12, the bacteria in the intestinal tract makes it for us by consuming fresh, natural plant foods, fruits, nuts, and seeds. The problem is the failure of proper digestion and absorption of foods because of our poor diets." - *Dr. Virginia Vetrano*

We do indeed make our own supply in our intestines, but once it has passed through the colon and ends up in the lower part of the "Ileum" it cannot be absorbed. I believe this to be partially true. Some experts claim that we have to eat our own feces to access our own B12, but clearly, we are not going to do this. In conclusion, when you do produce it by eating real foods, like we all naturally should, and are predisposed to absorb it, you will maintain your levels naturally.

Still, when you are a beautiful Vegan already for over five years (*estimate*), you could be at risk when living your animal free lifestyle with the criteria on page 198 (*A to E*). Because also Vegans can have poor digestion and an imbalanced intestinal flora when they eat little fresh produce with their meals to counterbalance the body's acid state (*all cooked foods produce an acid reaction*). Plus, the salt, sugar, spices, soy, grains, sodas, alcohol, and other irritants/non-foods can upset the bacteria family, so you need to be careful.

For this reason, you will have to be safe and protect yourself by,—*B12 supplementation*. It is something I do as well when taken out of the natural jungle and placed in a concrete one to be sure. I do not believe in supplements, but in this case, I do make an exception, as again, this is an extremely complex vitamin that needs to be respected. You can opt for injections or oral intakes that you dissolve under the tongue. Do not rely on the B12 fortified foods on the market these days as I do not trust its viability. Make sure that you supplement with the *superior form* of B12, which is the "Methylcobalamin." There are endless debates on which form is better based on its absorption and retention rate. Limited research is available, but I always choose the natural version over a cheap chemical copy that is *Cyanocobalamin*.

When testing for any deficiency, make sure you go for the "Methylmalonic" acid test, which is presently considered the *gold* standard for testing. Always keep in mind that this minor inconvenience of supplementing is an essential nuisance as the consequences of resorting to an animal diet, just for this vitamin, are far worse (*but you know this now*).

As you can imagine, there are many other important nutrients and vitamins besides B12 essential for health to talk about. Like, the importance of *Choline* and *Biotin* and many others, but this book would double in size. It suffices to know that your body will receive all its required nutrition when consuming a variety of fruits, veggies, dark greens, and small amounts of nuts and seeds. Be more alarmed by consuming dead foods and get caught in a perpetual loop of endless eating and poor nutrition, as was made clear in this book.

Can a Vegan diet improve a person's sex life?

When it is mostly raw and low fat, YES! Occasionally, I get this question, but indirectly. Mostly women will hint that their partner could use some help, as things are on a low flame. It is a very important inquiry as it plays an essential role in most relationships. The secret to your amazing machine's proper functioning is obviously the blood flow, as blood needs to be pumped throughout the body. It is no different with the sex organs. They rely on constant flow and pressure to function.

High blood pressure or "hypertension" though, can weaken the ability to increase blood flow to achieve an erection with men. Of course, when on the mainstream medical route, a prescription for a hypertension drug gets written, which often can result in a more poorly functioning organ. And that's why I will, as always, recommend to stay away from these drugs and focus on your diet.

A caution to all men is to be very careful when using the famous remedy,—Viagra. To think that you can reverse one bad drug effect (*if you are taking a hypertension drug*) with another is dangerous. Either way, a blue pill is not the answer.

All the body functions rely on the *biochemical laws* that govern them, so when breaking and disrespecting these laws, you are asking for trouble. Eat naturally, and exercise to run an efficient reliably machine that will never disappoint you, not even when "Cupid" calls.

It is a lot more complex with women as a dysfunction can have different root causes, but the remedy is pretty much the same. Respect your body and its infinite wisdom. Listen to its natural cycles that talk more clearly with a raw alive diet.

So again, "Yes!" Your sex life will improve when you follow your original design. When reaching your golden age, e.g., does not mean that this particular pleasure is not for you anymore. People often feel that their *age* is the prominent reason why things are not functioning as well as they used to, but this is not necessarily the cause. It is the decades of abuse through poor diet, alcohol, drugs, stress, etc. We are much better designed than that. So eat your fruits, nuts, seeds, and greens that will support you in those moments of passion. It is all natural healthy fun, so no need to be embarrassed.

What is the cause of constipation, is it dangerous, and what can I do to help it?

I sometimes feel that the whole world is constipated, as I learned that soo many people are suffering from it. As I mentioned before, true health starts in the colon, and thus we need to have more respect for our digestive system.

In the 1800s, sanatoriums were already bringing this awareness to the masses, like the famous "Battle Creek" of Dr. Kellogg (*yes, the inventor of the cornflakes*). These NH pioneers were already ahead of their time treating chronic conditions with, *Vegetarianism, exercise, enemas, fiber-rich foods, rest, pure water,* and *sunshine.* They are now replaced by wellness spas that offer massages and beauty treatments and a watered-down health approach.

What is devious to me is that these healing concepts that were there to really help a sick individual through natural ways did not become mainstream. They would have stopped the growth of massive hospitals as people would have been educated in a preventative lifestyle. It is obvious to me that somewhere it was decided that these natural practices were too successful in curing people. Also, because of no need for medications, they felt that NO MONEY can be made from disease! So, they were gradually closed to make way for large hospitals and their pharmaceutical partners in crime.

So, the key to real colon health, besides a diet of sufficient natural fibers, is fast digestion and exit. Any type of food that lingers too long will not only stagnate the digestion but also start the process of decomposition that inevitably leads to discomfort and ill-conditions,—even death in severe cases.

When the foods consumed, have none or very low water and fiber content, the needed support for quick passage is absent. Then it becomes abundantly clear why people suffer from constipation. Therefore, it is crucial that this is corrected once you know that you are constipated. Alarm bells should be ringing once you are aware that you have not seen your bathroom's interior for a while. Also here, the remedy is simple. STOP eating JUNK! START consuming REAL foods, as you learned in this book.

Let's not forget medications, especially pain drugs, as they are well-known causes of constipation, so do not resort to them too fast. A special caution here is needed to the use of "laxatives." The worst thing to do is to assist your *blockage* with a chemical laxative (*very toxic indeed*), which can turn things from bad to worse, especially when they have created a dependency. Clearly, it will be better to use natural remedies, like aloe vera, chia, flax seeds, coconut water, prunes, and other high fiber foods. The results on the body will be more gentle. But when you rely on these natural foods only in times of need, you still have to adjust your diet lifestyle. As also with constipation, preventing is preferred to curing.

The whole "peristaltic motion" that moves your waste out of your system is essentially a muscle that needs to stay trained. It is like breathing, a natural rhythm of the body that works only when given the right conditions. It thrives on fruits and veggies, low stress, proper food-combining, and exercise. So, to sum it up, you do not have to do anything but give it the foods it can work with that are natural. Another caution here is the use of "enemas" and "colonics" (*colonics are more thorough*). They can be helpful, but can also lazy, like laxatives, the peristaltic muscle, so do not overuse them. If you follow my guidelines, you will see that your trips to the bathroom will be frequent, fast, and rewarding.

The debilitating chronic conditions on the next page are becoming more and more widespread. These imbalances are the result of a wrong lifestyle, as pointed out. When we steer away from our original foods, our natural "defenses" become challenged. And after years of prolonged abuse, the body's protective barriers become weakened and falter. These three bowel and stomach related conditions serve as a warning to treat your digestive system with more love. Because you do not want to find yourself diagnosed with any of these!

I would like to put here an old "myth" at rest, which is that bananas promote constipation. If anything, they do the exact opposite, so please do not fear your yellow friend when in need of *movement*, *energy*, *nutrition*, and *detoxification*.

Leaky Gut, IBS, and Crohn's Disease

Leaky Gut	Our intestinal lining becomes compromised. This protective barrier controls what gets absorbed into the bloodstream. An imbalance may point to cracks or holes, allowing digested and undigested foods, plus toxic particles, to penetrate the walls. The body reacts with an inflammation to ward off the intruders.
IBS (irritable bowel syndrome)	This condition of the digestive system is the most unpleasant one. Bloating, gas, stomach cramps, diarrhea, and constipation are the fun effects you will have to deal with. They can plague you several days or even much longer. A correction of your lifestyle is needed.
Crohn's Disease	Inflammation in the bowels is the recognizable factor to this debilitating condition. Many similar symptoms as with IBS, but with more intensity and issues, like fatigue and weight-loss, together with bloody stools and mouth sores. Serious life-threatening complications can follow if no diet adjustments are taken.

What is candida, and how do I treat it?

The candida organism is found naturally in the healthy gut and intestines, skin, and mucous membranes. And as long as there is an equilibrium, they are your friends that keep things in check. Candida microorganisms work as a backup. When the blood's overall sugar levels increase to worrying levels, the candida starts consuming the excess to prevent a buildup.

This possible alarming situation can also extend to the pancreas and insulin production that cannot keep up with the amount of sugars in the diet. A high processed fat diet (*a very high natural fat intake can also be blamed*) is the culprit here as the fat molecules in the blood obstruct the sugar's delivery to the cells. Hence, an overgrowth occurs. Candida is also a precursor to many other maladies, so when in doubt, please see your MD to get tested.

- IBS
- Diarrhea
- Brain Fog
- Depression
- Jock Itch
- Chronic Fatigue
- Autoimmunity
- Constipation
- Migraines
- Eczema
- Psoriasis
- Ringworm
- Weight-gain
- Leaky Gut

As you remember from the *sugar step*, the consumption of processed sugars needs to be kept in control, together with our fat intake (*I will not stop mentioning this*). And these should only be consumed in its natural unprocessed form, like mangoes and avocados.

Another reason an overgrowth of candida occurs is the use of "antibiotics" (*prescription or food*). Its intake promotes the killing of good bacteria and onsetting an imbalance in our natural gut flora. This is another very crucial reason not to consume animal products as these creatures are routinely given antibiotics that get passed on to the consumer.

Then we have the other causes, like birth control pills, pain killer medication, and alcohol, to set this imbalance in motion. When dealing with candida, the goal is to reestablish the balance in your system by removing the sugar and fat. The idea is not to completely remove all the candida as you need it for health, just the excess. Natural sugar is not your enemy, but the strategy is to really lessen its intake and consume more greens than anything else for the time being. Any fat consumption will also need to be halted in the first stages of rebalancing. I assume that I do not need to emphasize the avoidance of alcohol and medications, if possible, in any way.

Once your candida levels are normal again, you can go back to eating fruits and fats, but the fat, of course, in small amounts and only the natural unheated ones and with the last meal of the day. "Did I mention this before?" Just kidding!

When going through any type of chronic condition that throws off your beautiful health, you will be reminded again that you just cannot eat everything that your eyes feast on and pleases your palate. Your body is incredible, but it has its limitations. It is not designed to be a "dead food" trash bin.

There are many different diet practices, and they all claim to be the one to follow. Why should I believe you?

I'll answer the last part first. It is not about believing me as I am only the messenger! Natural Hygiene is as old as life itself. Biochemical laws were in place when life came to be! Let me ask you: "How can nature herself not be the only path to follow?" Many diet fads are made up and fabricated by an individual to sell books. They create a new niche that fits the present market and trends and happens to work for some who try it, but it does not mean it will continue to do so in the long run. NH is different that way. It is like the manual that is included when buying a new car, if you get my meaning.

Lets review now the "pros and cons" of four popular diet crazes. As you will see, they all still lack crucial ingredients for pristine health and the well-being of our planet.

Macrobiotic Diet

Philosophy

We need to create a food balance through the teachings of "Yin & Yang." Grains are the staple and balanced with vegetables and soy. Grains are humanity's primary food, and we have to maintain our evolutionary status. We need to grow our foods in the area we live in. Eat local and organic!

Pros	Cons	
> Fruits and veggies > Nuts and seeds > No meat and fish > No dairy	> Soy products > Grains / pulses > Wheat products > Very high sodium > Malts and syrups	> Sea vegetables > Fruits cooked

Mediterranean Diet

Philosophy

Based on the atmospheric lives around the Mediterranean nations. The emphasis is on vegetables, fruits, grains, legumes, pulses, and fish like salmon, to substitute for the poor saturated fats, like cheese. Longevity is claimed, weight-loss, cardiovascular health, and an improved digestive system.

Pros	Cons
> Vegetables > Fruits > Nuts and Seeds > No refined oils	> Grains > Bread > Fatty fish > Dairy > Eggs > Some white and red meat

Keto Diet

Philosophy

Was initially developed as a treatment plan for pediatric epilepsy in the 20th century. Manipulates your body into Ketosis! A low-carb, high-fat diet, similar to the Atkins philosophy. By depleting the body of carbohydrates, which is its primary energy source, you force the body to burn fat for fuel. Primarily for weight-loss.

Pros	Cons
> No added sugars > Some veggies > Some nuts	> Meat and bacon > Fatty fish > Butter, cheese, and eggs > Use of much oil is encouraged > No fruits

Paleo Diet

Philosophy

The paleo or caveman diet believes that the processed foods we have been eating have only been around for the last one hundred years and agriculture for some ten thousand. We focus on eating nutrient-dense, whole, unprocessed foods that your body can digest easily and perform its best on, as nature intended.

Pros	Cons
> Fruits and veggies > Nuts and seeds > No grains and legumes > No processed foods > No dairy	> Raw and cooked meats > Fish and seafood > Eggs

Comment: If paleo dieters could agree that because meat has zero water and fiber and our own stomachs gastric acid secretions are far too low, efficient and complete digestion is impaired. Conclusion, we just cannot digest animal muscle (*our system cannot even handle seeds when swallowed whole, but I feel it is designed this way, so when pooping out the seeds, they will sprout new life, and so food*).

Plus, they need to recognize that meat and all fish are too fat. We have to stay out of the oceans as it is not the source for our food and its delicate Ecosystem needs to be protected!

Are all bacteria harmful? How do I safeguard my children from bacteria and viruses? I do not want them to get sick.

At the time of writing, the world is plagued by the "Covid19" virus, which resulted in the dramatic "Corona" pandemic! And like with all viruses, it will have to run its course until its last victim falls (*but it could return in more waves and also visit us every year as with the flu,—time will tell*).

Our history has given us quite the body count (*e.g. Spanish flu, 1918, ± 80 million dead*), and despite mankind's progress in medicine, we are still no match to these global outbreaks (*we could have been better prepared though, as experts did warn us after SARS, H1N1, and MERS!*). And these viral mutations will keep on coming if we do not change some fundamental hygienic protocols. Some information here on this Coronavirus will surely become outdated, even incorrect maybe. But there is one TRUTH that runs like a "deadly line" through all these outbreaks over history.

"Animal husbandry is an unnatural practice that manifests disease"

Ever since we started to stack up our housing structures and so creating a high population density within a certain radius while destroying nature's intricate fabric around it, we created unnatural living habitats. And these can only bring unhygienic problems! Today's mega-cities are the end result of this fiasco, and we need to rethink our infrastructures.

Up until the last century, human civilizations were still learning about personal and public hygiene, and we have come a long way. But not far enough, as we continue creating ideal breeding grounds for vermin and pestilence to flourish. Their presence goes on to threaten our well-being if we do not stay on top of it by endless exterminating and disinfecting.

We learned that us living in too close proximity to livestock is dangerous for our health together with the pests that once overran our streets and homes (*many are forced underground now and into the walls of our homes*).

Presently, there are many theories about how this pandemic started. Who is to blame, and how we can prevent this from happening again. To me, it has always been clear.

The following scene outplays in many parts of the world where animals are being handled. We still see markets where, legally and illegally, creatures of various species are caged in terrible filthy conditions and sold, traded, and eaten. Street dogs roaming around these markets together with rats, fleas, cockroaches, and other pests, creating dangerous "hotspots" for diseases and crossover mutations. I have seen the footage and these conditions in real life. You do not have to be a scientist or virologist to know that these condensed viral conditions are dangerous and need to be stopped!

But the world is hesitantly awakening to this hypothesis that animal consumption and wet markets are causing these unnatural mutations and endangering global health. I have already read the scientific reports of independent researchers that have concluded the same theory. Even the well-known "Peta" organization has now, in the aftermath of the pandemic, come out with a controversial (*it always is*) ad campaign:

"*Tofu did not cause a pandemic!*"

When you see people munching on the wings of a fried bat, that by the way, is once again being blamed for transporting viruses, you just know that it is very wrong. It is not easy to convince some traditional cultures that the eating of certain animal parts does not benefit your health nor your sex life!

Your immune arsenal will do the best it can, but when you abuse your body by creating a straining "obese" system, you just cannot expect it to work 100%. It has already been mentioned in the news that overweight people and/or an underlying chronic condition, like diabetes, have a greater risk of contracting ANY type of virus. Also, even though most people have learned that it is a respiratory condition, many still puff away on cigarettes and vape pens.

What will it take to smarten up? I hope that the public will now take this mask-wearing society as a message to improve their lifestyle and diet (*unrealistic hope, but hey*).

But besides blaming dangerous virus mutations at animal markets, we are dealing with a natural phenomenon that we face every year. I have learned and believe that the world this year (*2020*) is/was not on the brink of a very dangerous, deadly, and contagious disease.

Before the official pandemic lockdown, we were already underway processing an otherwise normal infection wave, with a mixture of different flu-viruses. And somewhere in there were/are the Corona strains. A whole lot of people were already carrying it for many months, and the explanation for the exponential growth in "cases" is the exponential numbers in "tests" conducted! This brought to light the many already infected people and causing the alarm. And what will make it likely come to an end, like every year? Weather. Atmospheric circumstances, like humidity, temperature, and upper currents, plus the growing immunity that makes it harder to spread.

This Corona kills, make no mistake about it, but also many people die yearly "world over" of the regular flu (*650.000*), tuberculosis (*1.5 million*), and heart disease (*about 8 million*).

I thought enough was said about this virus, but I kept on feeling that something was missing. Then, a friend sends me a link to a most fascinating guy who turns out to be holding the same bible as me. The "scripture" to respect Mother Nature, clean up our soils, and combat worldwide pollution.

His name is Dr. Zach Bush, MD. Triple board-certified in Internal Medicine, Endocrinology, and Metabolism. His view on this virus's cause is most intriguing and far from our mainstream info, and exactly what was missing here. When asked what a virus is, this was his response, quote:

*"**Viruses are a communication network of 'genomics' and the most important building blocks for life on Earth, and we have 'vilified' the very mechanism by which biology has happened on this planet!**"*

Unquote. He goes on to say that scientists and physicians are allowing the "demonization" of nature! They have now created the belief that these viruses are attacking us. Dr. Bush:

*"**Viruses are packages of information secreted by living organisms. They are the 'templates' for life**"*

He says that there is not enough genetic information in a single virus to do us any harm. Otherwise, viruses would have killed us all long ago! The point that he is getting to, that he is sharing with the world is, quote:

"This is a genetic 'update' to our species that's expressing an adaptation to the stress we've induced on the planet"

Unquote. Viruses were already around on the planet long before any animal was ever breathing. They were building the fabric of life from fungi and plants. They were constructing the complexity and diversity of life within the genetic code of the planet itself. He is so right in stating that science has such a narcissistic world view. That we are endlessly trying to make biology fit to us. I believe that there are always forces at work that cannot be analyzed nor seen under a microscope.

This Coronavirus attacks a HT receptor (*updating process*) in our lungs vascular tree and also the rest of the cells to make sure it gets delivered to the right ones to bring nature's genetic information into those cells. This process is a very intelligent distribution system and not in any way random.

All mammals were being updated, not just us humans. But reports of animals getting infected are very low. They do not suffer the same cardiovascular and metabolic diseases as we do. Our messed-up biology, due to wrong living in a toxic environment, has weakened humanity in many ways.

In other words, we are destroying our natural world with man-made chemicals for greed and so-called progress. We are now experiencing the effects of this foolishness through the chemicalization of our food system and the destruction of our soil by products like Monsanto's Roundup. We are destroying the important "homeostasis" of this virus and our "genome."

And together with our air and water pollution, we have all the ingredients for disaster.

He concluded his lecture by stressing that we need to: "Clean up our act!" As brought to your attention in this book. His detailed account of this intriguing insight into what the world is facing is needed to watch in full. So please look him up and become informed of what we are dealing with because I, for one, am not buying the government explanation.

But whatever caused this world's shutdown, we will pay the price for many years to come. I believe that we will never really know what happened or is happening.

Why does YouTube delete the videos where our doctors inform the public that Covid deaths are being inflated and that something is up? Sweden's strategy worked, as it has now (*October 2020*) falling numbers after their initial spike while other countries are preparing for a second lockdown! So, then why are no other nations adopting Sweden's no-mask rules and recognize that mostly the sick and elderly are vulnerable? There are plenty more controversies to explore, but I do not want this to become a "conspiracy" book.

My message, despite all this confusion, stays the same: "Take care of your beautiful health and support it the best you can for a happy and fulfilling life." There are no excuses anymore, as you have the manual right now in your hands!

And to answer the first part of the question. We live in a symbiotic relationship with all bacteria, and they are not a real risk for disease, as is believed by many (*only infectious bacteria*). Maintaining a clean alkaline system is crucial. As an acid one is the perfect breeding ground for bad bacteria to flourish. Please do not overwash your organic produce and be careful in using bleach and other *anti-bacterial* products.

Do not panic if your kids come home all dirty from playing outside, as it is still true what they say: "What doesn't kill you makes you stronger!" Just maintain a normal personal hygiene level to build a strong defense to the many microbes in our lives, and don't be too compulsive.

Why do you eat so strict, and what is your motivation for this lifestyle? It seems so boring.

(*People ask this question because my lifestyle puzzles them as I fall soo far from the norm. I hope that the following answer will motivate you to consider this new exciting direction*).

A lot of people just feel that life needs to be enjoyed, and I wholeheartedly agree. But, by not eating the delicious foods that the culinary world offers, it is perceived as "not enjoying life," strangely enough. Besides being unaware of the link between *health* and *food*, I feel this to be the basis for the question. Also, a healthy person, like a Vegan, is often seen as a threat to their lifestyle, a wake-up call, and many do not want to be awoken from their food addictions.

As I explained at the beginning of this book, information will set you "free!" Once you have explored the topic of food and health, you will see that they are intricately connected. And intertwined, we find LOVE. I do love life and myself being healthy in it, so it becomes then for me a logical action to adhere to nature's laws as explored in this book.

Mixed in with all this, you'll also need a decent dose of "rebelism," as you are going against the mainstream of social behaviors. "Dare to be different" is my motto!

Because at the end of the day, it is "You" who has to take care of yourself, and it is "You" who will be seeing the doctor when not well. And it is also "You" who has to face all the fear when waiting for a *heart bypass* or *cancer treatment*. I am sorry, but I'll pass on those. Of course, there are never any guarantees. But you can prevent many unpleasantries from taking hold of you in today's challenging world. We are being influenced to live a life that suits the powers that be! Don't jeopardize your beautiful health and happiness.

Every time I am in a supermarket, and I see those trolleys fully stocked, I need to bite my tongue to not point out the waste of money on these lifeless foods/products that people buy and could land you in that hospital. It is unimaginable the money we could save when not buying all these pointless items. We could then really enjoy life,—like more vacations.

What is boring? To a lot of people, it is the eating of pretty much only fruits, greens, and some nuts and seeds. At first glance, it maybe is, but most people do not have a clue about what is possible these days in the raw food kitchen. There are plenty of creations that you can enjoy that will bring variety to your plate. There is really no reason to get bored.

A new belief system is essential to be able to create a path of renewed health that will eventually become your truth. Then, you guard it against intruders. Seek out others for support and to help you maintain this rewarding lifestyle so that together we can all start to really evolve.

"Behold the power that resides in your original design, as we are the creators"

* * * * * *

NOTES

www.ingramcontent.com/pod-product-compliance
Lightning Source LLC
Chambersburg PA
CBHW032251150426
43195CB00008BA/412